Frozen Identity

Frozen Identity

K.Lee Black

ISBN 1-59109-974-9

To order additional copies, please contact us.
BookSurge, LLC
www.booksurge.com
1-866-308-6235
orders@booksurge.com

Frozen Identity

I would like to dedicate this novel to my two jewels,
Whitney and Madison.

ONE

The doctors and nurses stood perplexed, staring at the tiny imperfect human, wondering how such a freak of nature was allowed to complete the human gestation period. The skin, so white and transparent, granted views of the underlying dysfunctional systems. The eyes were blank, pink and unable to see the commotion they were causing. Albinism, the blatant defect in the infant, was joined by a host of flawed recessive genes. According to the bleak prognosis, the struggling soul was unlikely to survive the day of its birth. Genetic tests would supply some much needed answers. The baby's mother, fully conscious yet slightly groggy, lay on her back while the doctors finished suturing. Her blank stare led them all to believe that she was in shock. Her arms were bound tightly to the bed's side rails, a procedure that became necessary fifteen minutes ago during her hysterical outburst. Who could blame her? Expecting a beautiful, healthy, bouncing baby and giving birth to a grave deformation. The entire maternity wing couldn't help but hear the screams and accusations. The echo of, "Why my baby?" seemed to linger in the halls. When the nurses had attempted to take the infant to intensive care, the mother tried to follow. This was, of course, when they were forced to tie her down. The father of the baby, pacing in the waiting room, aware of only the emergency C-section, was anxiously awaiting the good news. He was confident his wife and baby were in the best of hands. Thirty minutes had passed since the medical team had shuffled him out of their way, to a soundproof, sparsely furnished room. The heat was blaring and so, it seemed, was background elevator music. Maybe something had gone wrong.

Both he and his wife had known that the sight of blood caused him to vomit, but maybe he was wrong to leave her side. He took reassurance in the words Amanda repeatedly stated about planting himself in the waiting room, in the case of any bloody complications. He was alone; finally he opted to sit as the fourteen hours of labor had taken its toll.

Slumped in the chair closest to the doorway, he found momentary refuge in his fixation on the cheap but rather soothing print hanging on the wall across from him. It was a watercolor filled with all the pastel colors that pleased his eye. His eye, of course, had been developed and fine-tuned by Amanda. Two years of marriage to an interior designer had done wonders for his sense of color, texture and balance. Their Sausalito condo, filled with pastels, emphasizing seafoam green, had always given his buddies ammunition for heckling. He was never offended, but routinely pretended to be annoyed at their sarcastic comments. Any one of them would gladly trade places, given the opportunity.

The print brought him back to the first day he had laid eyes on Amanda. The watercolored coastal scene before his eyes was almost identical to that early June morning. The similarity in the low lying shrubs and foaming blue-green water brought back the invigoration he felt as he followed her toward Stinson Beach. The sand dunes in the print were sculpted by the wind and formed a beautiful backdrop. The clever artist gave the viewer an opportunity to imagine the salty sea air and warmth of the beach, bringing life and therapeutic value to a once blank canvas.

TWO

Three Years *Earlier*

The energy, excitement and nervousness could be felt by persons not even involved in the race. The town square was running rampant with active metabolic tissue ready to erupt for eight miles across the treacherous mountain trails to take splendor with a dip in the ocean at the finish. Thus giving the race the name Dipsea. The quaint Northern California city just north of San Francisco nestled at the base of Mount Tamalpais was bustling with activity. The finish line at the Pacific Ocean, Stinson Beach, also drew an early morning crowd who busied themselves with setting up picnics for the arrival of friends and loved ones. The race started in Mill Valley. Eric's success in last year's race had given him the opportunity to run with the invitational runners. Invitational status was an honor given to those who placed in the first six to seven hundred the previous year, and thus were invited back the following year. Since handicaps were used heavily, women and children were fair game for victory. A team of exercise physiologists had tested the physiological capabilities at all ages, then staggered the runners accordingly. Eric was placed in the "scratch" section because of his age and sex. "Scratch" meant that all other runners with the exception of other "scratchers," had the advantage of starting before his section, thus giving the optimum challenge to these individuals. Women, children and males over thirty were placed in designated sections A-Y, and started their trek to Stinson Beach ahead of his section. The twenty-two minute delay wasn't supposed to intimidate him. After all, he was an under-thirty male whose muscle capacity and sheer strength should easily surpass the youngsters, the aged, and the weaker sex. Maybe if he repeated this ten times he'd begin to believe it.

Looking through the crowd he noticed the older men and young children gathering in the roped off "bullpen" which held only those runners who were next to begin their trek through Muir Woods to Stinson Beach. The race itself began eighty some-odd years ago and some of these old men in section A looked as if they could have run the original race. Most of them were great-grandfathers and would probably hit the century mark. Their frail appearance was sometimes deceiving. Often they were among the most competitive of opponents. The kids belonging to this section were eight and under, and a breed of their own. Born with the desire for challenge, speed, and pain, they are tough to beat and many finish in the top hundred. No amount of coaxing could have taken Eric away from his tree fort, rock collection or spit wad making at that age. Discipline came later.

After watching the first few sections start, Eric decided to take the next twenty something minutes for warm-up. His anxiety began to rise as race time neared. The lines for the outhouses were ridiculous, so after watering the bush behind the bus stop, a semi-private location that didn't bother him a bit, he began to jog around the square. As he began to feel warm, he met up with Mike, who was notoriously late and stooped over next to his car pinning on his number.

"So you thought you'd join us today, Mikey?"

Mike looked up and presented dark circles and puffiness around his eyes. When he spoke, he about knocked Eric over with his "hangover" breath.

"It was this irresistible girl I met at the carbo-load dinner. She was an animal, I tell you! I just couldn't pass it up.... or down. Mike's tongue movement accentuated his point while his devious smile filled in the gaps regarding the apparently fabulous sex the night before. His dark features contrasted beautifully against his perfect white teeth and deep green eyes.

His insatiable appetite for women was met and satisfied by the female masses who were equally hungry for him.

"I thought your bedpost had taken all the notches it could stand!"

"You are so jealous, Eric. Do you know where I could get some water? She drained me of all my bodily fluids!" He spoke casually and matter-of-factly, as if discussing an upcoming trial with a fellow lawyer.

"You look like shit. Why don't you stretch a bit and join me for a jog around the square?"

Eric began stretching his calves by leaning on Mike's brand new BMW, fully aware that fingerprints on his car was at the top of Mike's list of pet-peeves.

"I think I saw a Calistoga water stand set up near the start." Mike's eyes quickly analyzed the minute smudges, barely visible to the naked eye. Eric smiled.

Mike followed Eric's lead. Two loops around the square were sufficient, preceded by a five minute stretch and a gulp of water for Mike. After approaching the "bullpen" the third time they couldn't help but notice the rather large section gathering: Section "Q." The vast majority were women, very strong and intimidating. Most of the women required a second glance to verify their gender and some were so gaunt you wondered where they would find the energy to conquer such a grueling race. Eric and Mike quickly categorized the section into three groups: the "underweight obsessives," the "bull-dykes" and two women who fit their definition of "attractive".

One in particular sparked Eric's interest. Her body was slim and sculpted, with long graceful muscles. Unlike most women runners, this one had some curves. Her breasts were far from voluptuous, but were very female in structure. Her hair was sandy blonde, similar to his own. It was tied in a pony tail high on her head, revealing a fresh, beautiful face. With the exception of a hint of lip color, not a stitch of makeup was evident or needed. Her features appeared to be Celtic with high cheekbones, light eyes and skin. He found himself mesmerized by her every move and didn't take his eyes off her until the section "Q" gun went off. He lost Mike in the crowds.

With an eight-minute head start, she had quite the advantage over him. His only goal was to catch her and run the remainder of the race together. She, of course, would fall madly in love with him and they would live happily ever after. To his surprise, in the midst of his fairytale, he found himself leading all "scratchers" as he approached the stairs. The wonders of adrenaline and testosterone never ceased to amaze him! Eric could take the pain—knowing she was ahead. As he began climbing the first set of almost seven hundred wooden stairs, he caught his first "body" from the section that had left a minute ahead of his. His brisk momentum began to slow, but he continued to pass many bodies on the numerous flights of stairs. Heavy breathing, spitting and the rumble of pounding Asics and Nikes echoed through the dense sloping landscape. This indeed was a special breed today. A breed not afraid of grasping for their physical thresholds.

It was usually at this point in the race that Eric questioned his sanity. So many less abusive things he could be doing and he chose this...?

Three grueling miles into the race with his heart rate holding at its maximum and still no sight of her. He blurred his eyes at the open landscape, since soon the race would travel back into the heavily wooded areas. She was nowhere in sight. His confidence and hope had begun to fade. Who was he trying to fool, thinking a farfetched fantasy could become reality?

He was now pulling strength from resources he didn't know existed. Another mile and a half and he'd be working on the downhills. He strained to hold his concentration. He neared the second water station but decided to skip it, getting ahead of at least thirty runners who, instead, chose re-hydration. Finally he began approaching and passing what he perceived to be runners from the "Q" section. This gave him renewed hope of catching her. And then he saw her.

Green shorts and a deeper green running top. Her feminine strides were accomplished with the grace and agility of an antelope. Narrowing the distance between them was not an easy task. The path allowed for a single-file stampede, leaving little opportunity to pass bodies. With a steep mountain to his right and a cliff to his left, his only option was dangerous but necessary.

Passing on the cliff side without losing his footing took some careful, deliberate maneuvering. Each person he passed motivated the next death-defying act, until finally nothing stood between them. With time to relax and rejuvenate, he became more aware of his body as a mortal entity. To his surprise he noticed blood dripping from his inner left ankle. The endorphins had masked the pain and the excess moisture was the only reason he noticed the wound.

The sweet smell of her sweat kept him within feet of her at all times. If she slowed down, so did he. The downhill allowed for unimaginable relief. The feeling of overtaking such a brutal physical challenge was absolutely exuberating. It was impossible to gauge where they were in the pack of fifteen hundred, but his optimistic guess put them in the top third. Eric, along with his unknowing companion, were passing opponents at every opportunity. He literally felt as though they were flying.

Cool sea breezes coupled with a view of the ocean formed a backdrop and filled him with life. He knew he was as close to nirvana as he'd ever come. Adrenaline kept him going at this incredible pace. It was at this point that he understood why he chose this challenge. He wanted to scream exhilarating phrases at the top of his lungs.

On two occasions "Scratch" runners passed on their left. She glanced when they passed by, giving Eric an instantaneous view of her delicate profile. Oh how he wanted to reach out and touch her face. Behind her is where he planned to stay. Nothing else mattered. He was mesmerized by her body, her stride and the texture of her hair. And then it happened...he really should have been paying closer attention to the stairs.

Stumbling down at least twelve stairs knocked him out of his trance. It all seemed to happen in slow motion. His only concern was to roll, as best he could, out of her way. He tumbled over a cluster of grey jagged rocks. Thank God for the thin layer of green moss, slippery but cushioning and helpful in reducing open wounds. Except for a damaged ego and some minor cuts and bruises, he was, amazingly, still intact. Eric lay spread-eagled at the foot of the stairs. As he was coming out of his daze, a hand reached out to help him to his feet. Eric looked up to find his eyes meeting hers. The charming blue-green sparklers looked even more alluring when he stared directly into them. His embarrassment was overridden by her touch and kindness.

"Are you O. K. ?" She spoke with a rather winded drawl.

"Oh, I'm fine. Just lost my footing, miss." As soon as "Miss" came out, Eric realized it was not only too polite under these circumstances, but carried a lot of assumptions. On the other hand, he didn't stutter or drool, and that he could be thankful for.

"My name is Amanda," she remarked, chuckling from his choice of words. Her face was animated and beautifully flushed as she spoke. "Thanks for stopping. Really, I'm O. K., Amanda. " He staggered to his feet, attempting to regain some sort of composure. Assured that he didn't need medical attention she continued down the mountain. As she disappeared into the thicket, he remembered that he had forgotten to introduce himself. Immediately, he cupped his hands to his scuffed-up face to carry his yell like a megaphone. "My name is Eric,. . Eric...Eric...Eric. . ," echoed down the mountain.

He stayed back to check the damage once again and blot the bleeding on his knee and forehead. Beautiful and compassionate, he thought as he gathered himself and began down the mountain.

It wasn't until the last mile that he caught a glimpse of her. She was toward the front of a large cluster of runners less than a quarter mile ahead. Catching her this time would be a bit more painstaking since his newly developed limp and throbbing head were a detriment to his pace. This time she got away.

Clear skies and soothing sun were a rarity at Stinson Beach at 10:00 AM in June. It was almost too warm to be finishing a twelve-kilometer race that began in the early morning fog of

Mill Valley. Eric had trained for months for this event. Initially, his goal was to finish in under an hour, five minutes faster than last year's time. With that accomplished, he began scanning the mob of runners and supporters. He knew as time went by that his chances of laying eyes on Amanda were quickly diminishing. The mob was growing dense as more runners finished. Exhausted runners clamored aboard the shuttle buses back to Mill Valley. Desperate, his eyes adhered to anyone resembling her. His legs brought him closer until he realized his attempts were futile. The aimless succession of failures lasted for quite some time.

Depressed and dehydrated, he walked toward the water station. An unusually strong headrush overtook him, and threw him off balance. The ground seemed to move from beneath him. For fear of falling he quickly crouched and placed his head between his legs. Before he could reorient and gain steadiness, a blur of bodies swarmed, an I.V. was inserted, a doctor shined a light in his eyes and the sound of ambulance siren was blaring. Reality was obscured and he wondered if he was dreaming, or simply lapsing into a distorted subconsciousness. A microphone was shoved in his face and a camera was pointed at his failing body.

At this point everything went black.

THREE

Eric smelled the sterile aroma and knew this wasn't a usual one-night stand. Opening his eyes confirmed this and instantly brought him back to Stinson. Slightly disoriented, he began looking around the small curtained area where he lay, hooked up to an I.V. along with two other high-tech contraptions. The "monitor" of sorts was checking his heart, which immediately increased when he noticed Amanda standing beside his bed.

"Do you always try to kill yourself twice a day, or is this behavior uncharacteristic?" As her words came out he was more interested in hearing her voice inflections and watching her sumptuous lips at work than in listening to the actual content.

She waited for a response but Eric was at a loss for words. "Oh, I guess the fluids haven't fully hydrated your brain yet," she commented as she sat and slid her chair closer to the bed.

Taking advantage of the situation, Eric continued to give her a blank stare. He knew he could get away with it in his pathetic condition. He noticed she was probably a few years older than he originally had thought and visible under these harsh lights were a few lines around her eyes and on her forehead. Her contoured cheekbones were not covered with a layer of supple flesh, common to women in their teens and twenties. This observation didn't detract a bit from her features and, in fact, gave her the sophisticated look he especially was attracted to. He guessed her age at thirty-two, or five years his senior. "Now you know my secret for getting attention! First, throw yourself down a cliff and, if all else fails, pass out in a crowded area, making sure, of course, that a news crew and an ambulance are nearby!"

They both broke into laughter. Eric was thrilled something halfway witty was allowed to escape his lips, a rarity for him when it came to virgin conversation with an attractive female. "Coolness" was almost unheard of in these instances.

Amanda had a great smile. One that allowed a glimpse of a great abundance of white teeth. The kind of smile that made the lucky recipient feel special.

"Well, I'm glad to see you're going to live. You were out for almost twenty minutes. I was really worried. I guess I'll let you get some rest. " Amanda began to rise.

"Wait just a cotton pickin' minute," he said, hoping to humor her again, and to detain her in the process. "You've gone beyond the call of duty twice today. You're not leaving until I thank you and think of a way to repay you." She abruptly sat, startled at Eric's comment.

Then she stood up, turned and faced Eric. She stared into his eyes. Eric prepared for some romantic overture. Instead, she said rather coyly, "Well, are you going to thank me now or is your brain on the fritz again?"

He calculated the behavior to be flirtatious. Whatever it was, he liked it. "I'm still confused about how I got here and how you ended up with me. Thanks so much for staying. What exactly happened after I passed out?" She began speaking and he strained to pay attention to the content. "A crowd was gathering around the water station," she began. "I assumed it was the first place finisher because the news crews were hovering. As I approached I saw people gathering around an injured man who was lying down. My first thought was that it might be Henry, so I rushed over to get a closer look. Who do I see, but the guy who tumbled down the stairs at 'Cardiac Hill.' I noticed as they placed you on the stretcher that there was no significant other," she continued as her face began to show a hint of embarrassment. "Well, I couldn't exactly let you ride in an ambulance alone. I simply told the medics that I was your sister. "

The curtains were pulled back and an elderly nurse began to poke and prod. "Glad to have you back with the living Eric.

I just can't understand kids nowadays." She turned towards Amanda for a fleeting moment and directly back towards her 'victim'. "In addition to killing themselves to climb the corporate ladders, they consider a ten-mile run relaxing. We worked hard in my day, but knew how to relax when the day was done," she continued without coming up for air. "All you athletic types are way too skinny if you ask me. I like a man I can dig my knuckles into. And look at your sister—just as skinny as a rail."

Finally the focus left Eric but returned when the rambling geezer began to fool with the tubing that allowed the slow trickle of fluids to replenish his dehydrated body. Eric was feeling exposed and uncomfortable as the nurse began prodding with her fingers, depressing his skin and waiting for the appropriate response. Embarrassed, Amanda looked elsewhere.

"You're practically a 'John Doe.' The only information we have is your first name. This is far from normal hospital procedure but with you out cold and your sister so upset, I convinced my supervisor to let it slide. Anyway, you look like the type to have health insurance. Do you feel up to answering some questions before I get fired?" The nurse was blunt, but evidence of a soft side was close to the surface. Amanda tried to hide her smile but let out a restricted laugh as Eric nodded in agreement. "Nurse Clooney"—Eric noticed her worn-out name tag—picked up the clipboard, adjusted her pen and began firing questions like a drill sergeant.

"Eric Edwards.... 576 Tam Junction Road.... . 555-5376." As he continued he realized Amanda, if interested, had all the information she needed to make a first move. Maybe she didn't have a problem with that, he thought hopefully.

"I really should be going now," Amanda said, "I'm sure Henry is worried sick."

Eric had no idea who Henry was, but noted her nervousness both times she talked of the fellow. It was then that he noticed the ring. Amanda couldn't miss the rush of astonishment glaring in Eric's eyes. "Is Henry still waiting at Stinson?"

"I know...I really shouldn't be here. I was just worried

about you, Eric. I couldn't let them take you to you hospital alone. Now that I see you're fine, I'll be leaving." As she turned to walk away, he said with all the hope he could muster in his tone, "Amanda...is there a law that says we can't be friends?"

"My last name is Black, as in the bruises on your ass." The door closed. She was gone.

Eric felt the weight of her stare and anticipated another lecture coming on from old Nurse Clooney. She opened with raised eyebrows and a devious smile.

"Quite a strange relationship you and your 'sister' have, wouldn't you say? It's really none of my business, Eric, but is there something I should know? That girl looks familiar. Maybe I can help. I thought I saw too much spark between you two for you to be simply siblings! You do love her, am I right?"

The woman had no limits. There was no end to her back-to-back questioning, and Eric saw she had no qualms about delving into the personal lives of others. He looked at Nurse Clooney, smiled, and closed his eyes.

Later, as he tried to sit up, the room began to spin. He could hear a humming sound and could see, through the sparkling dots floating in the air, Nurse Clooney's mouth flapping. He could feel the world going black again, but before the 'door' shut completely a strange odor made him come to. There stood Nurse Clooney, holding smelling salts below his nostrils.

"Well, Eric, it looks like they're planning to hold you overnight for observation. We just can't let you go until you're stable. The routine blood tests have been ordered, just in case."

"In case of what?" he mumbled.

For the first time, Nurse Clooney's grandmotherly professionalism began to slip. It was apparent she was nervous about something. "Well, it's probably just that you over-exerted yourself, which could account for some of the values being out of kilter."

"What values are you referring to? Let's not beat around the bush."

"When you were first admitted Eric, you were out cold. Your 'sister' was of no help with the family history. We felt it necessary to run some very routine blood tests. Some of the values were out of the normal range. It's probably nothing to worry about, but we need to rule out everything."

"Everything...you sound like you're suspecting an army of problems. Is there anything in particular that you suspect?" For the first time, his stomach began to turn.

"At this point, Eric, we wouldn't even attempt a guess. Without further medical tests we haven't a clue. It's probably nothing, like I said. Relax, get some rest and leave the rest to us. If you'd like to make a call, just dial nine and listen for a tone." She smiled and motioned toward the black high-tech telephone on the bedside table.

She left the room. The door was still ajar when she slipped her head back in.

"I almost forgot to tell you...You are famous. Channel Five has called three times. If you are feeling up to it, they'd like a short interview with you later this afternoon. "

Great, he thought. They plan to let the whole Bay Area know about the poor sap who passed out after the Dipsea.

As he lay in the sterile little room, he began to think about whom he should call. He decided to spare his parents from the unnecessary worry, couldn't get through to his vacationing boss and shared secretary, put the phone down and decided against contacting anyone. Eric was sure Mike would have a field day as soon as the news aired.

He closed his heavy eyes knowing Amanda would soon enter his dreams.

The news crew came knocking on his door, waking him just minutes into his much needed nap. After a small, rather reluctant nod on his part, before they began to set up shop. The cameraman and his assistant were literally in his face, trying to assess the exact focus and angle of operation. As they plugged in cords and lights they spoke under their breath about a mix-up at the hospital. Something about a wrong room and a guy on his deathbed. Nervous chuckles were followed by more talk about their relief that Marla was running behind and would never find out. They continued but their voices were no longer audible as they began to turn on the camera equipment.

Marla Dune of Channel Five evening news made her appearance in Eric's room fifteen minutes before air time. She looked much shorter in person. Without acknowledging Eric, she walked directly into the far corner of his less-than-expansive room. She pulled some notes from her briefcase and feverishly began reviewing.

"Do I have time to use the bathroom, or should I wait for the power surge first?" Eric sarcastically remarked.

Marla looked past her makeup person and for the first time caught eyes with her interviewee. By the look on her face, the comment had caught her off guard. Eric began to wish he could take it back. "I'm sorry Eric. We were told by the hospital to hurry the interview. I was running behind and surely didn't mean to slight you. Please take whatever time you need and we'll be out of here as soon as we can."

As he sat up in bed, he began to feel woozy. When the room stopped spinning he stood, walked toward the bathroom and made sure the flap in his hospital gown didn't expose his bare ass. The clock on the wall said five-twenty. His internal clock said two A.M. The bathroom mirror confirmed how he felt. He urinated, splashed water on his face, made an attempt to calm his unruly hair and shuffled back toward the bed. Now, more awake and hopefully looking more alive, he pushed the button to adjust the bed to the upright position.

Marla moved toward him with a confident gait. She looked much better in real life. He would almost venture to say she appeared attractive. Her red suit declared a fit body underneath. He wondered if Marla was a runner or possibly an 'aerobics queen.' Maybe she took this interview out of personal interest.

"Before we get started, Eric, I have a few questions. Do you mind?"

"No, not at all. I have a few of my own if you don't mind?" he said as he made an attempt at sitting more erect.

"O.K., was this your first year running the Dipsea?" Marla didn't hesitate to start the questioning.

"No, I ran it last year too."

"Do you think the heat had something to do with your passing out?"

"I'm sure it played a part, but I think dehydration was the major reason."

"Do you feel there should have been more water stations along the way?"

"That wasn't a problem. It was my pacer...This woman I tried to keep up with. Well, she never stopped for water. I liked her pace and didn't want to lose her. Then I took a tumble and lost her. I spent the next three miles playing catch-up. I guess I dehydrated myself in the process. The heat aggravated it, but definitely wasn't the cause."

"Am I correct in assuming that this woman—your pacer—accompanied you in the ambulance?" She raised her eyebrows.

"Yes, but what does that have to do with...?"

"She's Amanda Black, who came in second overall and was the first-place woman today. Were you aware of this?"

Eric's mouth hung open. His eyes felt as if they had disengaged from their sockets.

"This is an enormous upset...very unexpected. Cameras at the start of the race and along the way verify an honest victory. They also verify that you and Amanda were together for a couple miles approximately midway through the race. And then we lost track of you, until the finish after you lost consciousness. We're curious about your relationship with Amanda and anything you can tell us about her."

"I guess I was foolish to think my physical state was of any concern to you." Eric went back to his original notion that Marla Dune was only after a good story at the expense of others. Her brief attractiveness faded as she began to resemble a vulture.

"Marla, we're ready to roll whenever you are..."

Eric never did get to his questions that day.

∽♪∾

"Rise and shine, Eric. I see a night's rest is all you needed. Your color is back. Just to make sure, let's beat the rush to the lab." Nurse Clooney put the 'P' in pep as she scooted the wheelchair to his bedside.

"Why fight it, I know you won't take no for an answer." Eric couldn't help but like the old nurse.

The wounds on his knees had formed two huge scabs and his muscles were incredibly stiff. He welcomed the wheelchair. Before he could adjust the foot rests, they were cruising the hospital corridors towards the lab. The hospital aroma was making him queasy and the thought of another needle penetrating his flesh wasn't helping matters. A momentary glimpse of a man lying in his bed with tubes protruding from every available orifice pushed him over the edge. Dry heaves prompted his body to catapult itself to the floor. Nurse Clooney felt bad as she almost ran him over with the wheelchair. The episode, though brief, was embarrassing and humiliating. Kneeling and retching in the presence of a very ill man. Eric couldn't help but notice a banner hanging over the poor man's bed that read "Get Well Soon, Edward." Knowing the man's name made the imprint even deeper. The news crew must have seen Edward and assumed they were in Eric's room. He now understood the nervous chatter from last night's cameramen. What a dreadful mix-up.

FOUR

In the past few years, with the economy in somewhat of a slump, 'New Designs' had been forced to redirect its focus from individual to corporate design development. Henry had brought Amanda into the Tiburon based company eight years prior to the stagnating economy. Amanda was insecure, gorgeous and freshly graduated from a highly-accredited art school. Henry welcomed the challenge and opportunity and took her under his wing, showing her the 'ins and outs' of interior design, as well as business in the real world. Amanda was virtually swept off her feet by Henry's sophistication and distinguished appeal. Soon after, Amanda bought into the company and became Henry's partner. Two years later they were married. 'New Designs' had begun in Henry's garage twenty-six years ago and had become the leading design company in Northern California. His passion and innate sense of aesthetics kept the company thriving while competing companies failed. Amanda's talents added new dimensions and continued its success. Their close friends considered Amanda and Henry to have a perfect partnership in all senses of the word. The only exception was hidden. A secret to take to their graves.

Henry sat motionless at his desk, staring, as if in a trance, out his office window. The spectacular view encompassed at least seventy-five percent of the bay with a clear shot of the Golden Gate and the City. On a clear day it was almost possible to focus on the hustle-bustle of Fisherman's Wharf and the Embarcadero. The soft natural light made his grey hair shine and his blue eyes glisten. His strong jaw and lean muscular stature were those of a man much younger than his fifty-one years.

His numerous attempts to concentrate on the seventeen-page design contract sitting on his desk seemed futile. It was nearly noon, almost three and a half hours since his arrival, and like every Monday he would meet Amanda for their standing lunch date at 'Sam's.' The funky hang-out was a popular lunching spot for Tiburon's professionals and anyone, for that matter, having the desire to enjoy a relaxing meal on a boat dock. Stocked heavily with plastic tables and chairs, 'Sam's' could accommodate the lunch and dinner rush with ease. The waitresses, whose dresses were a size too small and a foot too short, obliged all the customers' needs. The atmosphere was the prevailing lure, making the food almost irrelevant.

Henry's anticipation was building. Ever since she abandoned him at the Dipsea yesterday, something was up with Amanda. Henry noticed her absolute preoccupation but hadn't a clue where her mind was wandering. Keeping his temper in check was difficult but ever so necessary after his last tantrum followed by Amanda's heated warning. He suspected she would follow through with her threat to leave if he ever laid a hand on her again.

His eyes were drawn to the clock at two minute intervals the entire morning. Finally, at ten to twelve he allowed himself to stand, stretch, put the phones on the service and make his way to the underground parking garage. His black Porsche 911 convertible had just been detailed, and it competed with its polished driver. The fog unveiled a cloudless blue sky on this predictable June day.

Insecure, Henry caught her eyes immediately, as she was escorted through the restaurant and past its dining patrons. The dock seating was packed. The sounds of laughter, casual conversation and glasses clinking in the bar were not only audible but dominated one's senses. The blue-green bay against the colorful harbor formed a beautiful backdrop for visual pleasure. Henry forced a smile to help relax the tension in his forehead. Amanda looked radiant in her scoop-neck linen dress.

Understated, simple lines with soft textures never competed with her beauty and delicate frame. Her shoulder-length, silky, ash-blonde hair was hanging naturally for the wind to move at will.

"Both early, as usual." Henry reached for his habitual embrace.

"That's why we make such a good team, Henry." She reciprocated half-heartedly.

"How was your meeting this morning, Amanda?"

"Challenging, but I think I won them over. I offered them a ten percent reduction if they sign by Friday and the CEO jumped on it. I figure I can make up for the loss on the build-out materials and labor."

"How was your morning?" She brushed her hands through her hair and thought of Eric.

"Far from productive, I must say." Henry could see she was drifting as he attempted to delve into the dark recesses of her mind. Worry and fear began to surface on Amanda's face, which to Henry's warped intuition appeared as guilt or deceit.

"What's on your mind? I feel like you're on another planet. Is it something I said? Ever since your disappearance after the race you haven't been yourself."

For the first time in nearly a decade Amanda spoke to Henry in half-truths. As she spoke she noticed that Henry's distinguished features began to look aged. She could clearly see his rage through his facade of calmness. Thoughts of deceit were made easier as memories of the back of his hand repeatedly striking her surfaced. The physical pain was healed, but the mental anguish remained.

"I think placing in the Dipsea has gone to my head. An egomaniac at age 31!" She said it with a smile. "Anyway, I wasn't the one who left his wife behind at Stinson. Thank God for the stash in my shoe to call a cab." The lie seemed to flow effortlessly from her mouth as she glanced occasionally over Henry's shoulder, in unrealistic hopes of seeing Eric. She wondered why he wasn't returning her call. She worried that he might still be in the hospital. "I waited for forty-five minutes and you were nowhere to be seen." He bit his lip. "See, you're doing it again, Amanda." Henry's voice began to rise to uncontrollable levels. "Who are you looking for anyway? Remember, young studs may look good on the outside. Their bankbooks paint a different picture. They can never provide for your happiness the way I do."

Amanda's appetite for lunch, and Henry, was quickly diminished. She began to look at her marriage differently. The remainder of the afternoon, in the same quarters with Henry, made Amanda feel almost claustrophobic. She left the office early to run some conjured-up domestic errands. Arriving home, she headed straight for the answering machine. Still no message from Eric.

Eric's impatience was building to the point of explosion. It was nearly noon and still no sign of the doctor. He looked once again at the clock and decided to leave with or without the results by one o'clock. Twenty-four hours in any hospital was one day too long.

With no appointments today and the ability to leave an appropriate message on the office machine via the hospital, Eric felt comfortable about missing work. Only three messages had come in since the weekend. The first was his business partner, Richard, calling from the Virgin Islands. Making Eric jealous was Richard's full intent of the call. After a long-winded description outlining his sailing expertise, suntan lotion-lubing contests and tropical drink consumption, he did ask how the 'rookie' was holding down the fort. Richard, a CPA for over twenty years, had a talent for relaxation and fun. Eric admired this attribute and hoped he would follow in his shoes.

The second message was from Mike. He apparently had received Eric's message from this morning and said he dropped off some clothes before work. Mike was a guy who always came through when the going got tough. Eric couldn't say that for too many lawyers, or people, for that matter.

Noticing the bag placed in the chair adjacent to the bed,

Eric opened the gym bag and smiled. Mike had packed his Valentine's boxer shorts covered with red and pink Cupids. His pink shirt and jock were also thrown in for laughs. Stuffed partially in the front hip pocket of his jeans was a note.

Hope all is well...wanted to make sure you look pretty and feel loved.

Mike finds humor in every situation and was always able to get a laugh out of Eric.

Don't forget to call after you talk to the doctor.

Below his signature the note continued...

We all know you're way too 'studley' to truly be sick!

The third message had been left by Amanda. He picked up the phone and started dialing her newly memorized number. A male voice answered and Eric, like a school boy, hung up immediately. His heart was pounding and his face turned red. The palms of his hands were moist.

After showering, he gathered his still damp and quite ripe running clothes, 'crusty' shoes and watch and stuffed them into his gym bag. He picked up the scrap containing the message Nurse Clooney had given him, practically obliterated from spending so much time in his sweaty, pondering hand. Hours of contemplation helped him to come to a decision which he planned to carry out after arriving home. He placed the note in his jeans, next to Mike's.

Dr. Ronald Branson entered Eric's room just shy of 1:00 ; two hours late. He brought with him a hematology report identifying the results of the tests and no apology for his tardiness. His skin appeared grey from lack of sunlight and physical exertion. He walked with a hesitant gait and reached to shake Eric's hand. His firm shake showed true dedication. He spoke simply, in laymen's terms, with no sign of arrogance. His voice was deep and full of compassion. He paused, swallowed and opened the conversation as Eric's anticipation grew.

"Hi, Eric, I'm Ron Branson, Chief of Hematology at Marin General. I have reviewed your blood work and I'm happy to bring you news of your near perfect health. You're slightly anemic, which an increase in your iron intake will eliminate. We hope you had a comfortable stay." He began scribbling something important on the pad he pulled from his breast pocket. "Supplementing your diet with 65mg of ferrous sulfate three times a day should do the trick. You'll find it at the pharmacy here or at your local drug store."

"Thank you, Doctor, I'm relieved to hear everything is O.K."

❧

The soothing morning sun and calm blue sky shone through the bay window of Amanda and Henry's sitting room. Henry sat with paper in hand, immersed in the business section. The expensive rattan chair with matching ottoman and end table formed a picture of relaxation. The table was clad with a crystal vase full of mixed flowers, a cappuccino in a finely crafted cup and two of John Steinbeck's masterpieces. Amanda sat on a small floral loveseat that was situated in the southern corner of the room, perpendicular to an expansive window. The diffused but warming light complemented her ivory skin. Excluding the tension, the scene could have made the cover of Better Homes and Gardens.

Appearances can be deceiving.

The Architectural Digest failed to impress Amanda this Tuesday morning. Nothing seemed to interest her except for Eric. She had too much pride to call him again and the waiting was excruciating. She and Henry would be leaving for work soon, and since they would be at the office all day, Henry had suggested they drive in together. Amanda's immediate response to the suggestion didn't sound concocted.

"I think a run to the office this morning will be just the thing for these tight gastronemiuses." She massaged her calves for effect.

Thank God, Henry let it go at that and eased up on the suffocation, for the time being anyway. Amanda began to feel confident in regard to thinking on her feet and guilty in regard to her mild deceit.

At eight-thirty, like clockwork, Henry walked to the kitchen, rinsed his cup and headed for the bathroom to tend to his oral hygiene in his usual meticulous manner. This ritual was at least a ten-minute ordeal, starting with a rinse of sorts, a thorough brushing with an electric contraption he had purchased through the Shopping Channel, and then a flossing of the crevices, followed by the gargling of mouthwash. When he was nearly finished Amanda walked to their bedroom and dressed in her jogging outfit. After seeing Henry off, she sat on the loveseat and stared at the phone, hoping it would ring. It didn't, and after ten minutes of testing a clairvoyant strategy she decided to turn on the stereo and warm-up to some Anita Baker. Her run to the office was relaxing and therapeutic.

With a clear mind and a better grasp of reality, she began to see Henry in a better light. Her morning with Henry was almost tolerable. She managed an apology and embraced him after seeing he had decorated the office in irises and tulips. Henry, with loads of work piled on his desk, thought it best to work through lunch. Amanda decided to lunch at home and bring back Henry's.

As she was turning the key on the patio french door, the phone began to ring. With her brisk, deliberate movement and experience with the lock, Amanda managed to pick up before the second ring was finished. Her heart rate rose and a cool sweat began almost instantaneously. There was no voice on the other end, but she knew it was Eric.

Amanda's appetite vanished. She forced down half of a turkey sandwich and packed the remainder for Henry, along with some leftover Chinese take-out, a Calistoga water and two jumbo chocolate chip cookies.

Eric's apartment was pretty standard. A couple of leather couches set in a predictable configuration, a few unimaginative prints, grey carpet with an occasional garment or towel tossed in a heap. Not a single wreath, flower arrangement or woman's delicate touch in sight. All in all it was decent and in a high-rent area, even for Marin. Greenbrae, an upscale community, housed many prominent doctors, lawyers and other professional people. Eric rented the ground floor of an expansive tri-level home owned by an eccentric old widow. The house had been paid off nearly two decades ago, and with her healthy savings and assets, combined with a $750,000 life insurance check, Mona Bixby was set. Mona's husband had passed away three years prior, leaving William, Mona's son, to fill his shoes as a partner at the fertility clinic he had operated. William spent the majority of his waking hours running the clinic and the minuscule remainder of time with his wife and two young children. Although their homes were separated by fewer than fifteen miles, Mona's visits were limited to holidays. She was lonely and thought of Eric as a surrogate son. Eric enjoyed Mona's company too, but originally moved in because the rent was reasonable and was reduced considerably in the months when he helped around the house—just about every month outside of tax season.

It was still early in the afternoon when Eric pulled into the driveway on Tamal Vista. Mona, kneeling as she tended to her roses and herbs, perked up from her slouch when his car door slammed

"I know I'm not your mother, but I've been worried sick. Mike was here early this morning, but he was gone by the time I put my robe on and went downstairs." Her face showed the strain Eric had put her through and the amount of concern she had for him. Eric felt as if he were seven again and had forgotten to say "thank you" to a grandparent after a day at the carnival.

"Mona, I know I should have called last night." Eric felt fine, but decided to play into her sympathetic soft spot. He put his eyes at half mast, slowed his speech and added a bit of a limp to his gait. He walked toward Mona and opened his arms for his usual greeting embrace. "Well, I felt lousy after waking up with all the needles stuck in my body. Exhaustion accounts for the rest of my excuse. I'm sorry, Mona. I don't blame you for being upset." Eric was absolutely sincere but omitted mentioning how his forgetfulness was directly related to the fact that he'd fallen in love.

Tears welled in Mona's eyes as they embraced. "You know I think of you as a son. What would I do without you? Let's go inside and talk about what happened. I made some strawberry shortcake and a new herb tea concoction for you to sample."

Mona peeled off her soiled gardening gloves and they walked hand in hand on the mossy brick path toward the house. Eric was forgiven.

At five-twenty two, alone at last, Eric dialed Amanda's number for the second time. The phone rang and before his nerve plummeted, a familiar voice answered.

"Hi, may I speak with Amanda Black?" He knew Amanda had picked up, but if he deviated from his prepared first sentence he'd probably stutter or freeze.

"Eric, is that you?" Amanda said nervously. "I can't talk now." She took an audible deep breath. "Can you meet me at slip #113 at the Sausalito Marina at eight?"

Before the question was transmitted to his brain, the phone went dead. Must be the home phone, Eric thought.

The sunset was magnificent with smeared purples, pinks and luminescent yellows and oranges. The wind had died down to a calm ocean breeze. Eric parked the Saab behind the mountain bike shop and debated if he should bring the wine and french bread he'd purchased at Cost Plus en route to Sausalito. Strawberry shortcake wasn't going to hold him until morning, but his stomach was in knots and he highly doubted it would improve once he was in Amanda's company.

His heart was racing as he neared the sailboats. Without a clue to where the slip numbers were located, he hunched to get a view of the front edge of the dock, as if he were checking the curb in a suburban neighborhood. From a distance he heard the same restrained laughter he remembered hearing yesterday afternoon. He turned. What he saw took his breath away. She wore a white gauze sundress and tan sandals. So simple, yet elegant and natural. Her smile spanned the width of her finely chiseled face. The light breeze combined with her graceful stride blew back her hair, exposing the elegance of a true beauty.

"I was giving it a fifty-fifty...I'm so glad you could make it." She was toting a bag of groceries. French bread baguettes, wine and fruit were visible and protruding from the sack; Eric was glad he had also packed some edibles. "I need to apologize for my brevity on the phone. You see...Henry was home and..."

Eric interrupted, "And where does he think you are now?"

"With my latest lover, of course. We've been married for almost a decade and he's been paranoid for the greater part of it. You may find it hard to believe, Eric, but you are the only man that I've met at the harbor. I've been completely loyal, and had no desire to do anything to the contrary." Amanda stared into the sunset. She continued with earnest seriousness. "Something happened yesterday. I noticed you before I began the race. I noticed you noticing me. Eric...I can't eat or sleep. My mind is occupied with thoughts of you." She looked at him and smiled. "You can chime in whenever you please or run the other way if you think I'm completely psychotic!" She began walking. Eric joined her and they strolled in sync to the last sailboat on the dock.

"I don't think you're crazy; maybe it's a bit risky to lie to your overprotective husband. I can't say I blame him for being a bit insecure. A gorgeous woman is definitely something to hold on to."

Amanda stopped, turned and reached for his hand as she stepped onto the magnificent boat. Her hand felt natural in his and didn't let go of the mutual grasp until they were 'under-cover' in the cabin of this yacht she called a sailboat. The woodwork gleamed beautifully and complemented the polished brass fixtures. The cabin was accented tastefully with nautical upholstery and appeared to be fully equipped with all modern conveniences.

He placed the groceries in the bar area. When he turned, she was within inches, looking straight into his eyes. Their emotions were in turmoil, and senses overstimulated. The beauty of the cabin, with quality workmanship abounding and this beautiful woman wanting him...It was almost more than he could stand. Their embraces were long and tender; they called upon their inner strength to control their desires. Conversation steamed from their mouths and laughter was frequent. Time passed quickly and nervousness filled the cabin as they drank wine and nibbled on bread and cheese. Thoughts of where the relationship was headed filled their minds and eventually left voids in the conversation, finally putting a close to the evening.

ᏬᎯᏫ

Henry stared out the window facing the drive that led to their home. It was close to 11:00 and his anger was on the verge of eruption. He'd been pacing for over an hour and was contemplating a drive to the aerobics studio when he spotted Amanda's Range Rover pulling up the drive. He gulped the remainder of his third martini and walked toward the kitchen to rinse, dry and carefully place the glass, and any other evidence of his drinking spree, out of sight. He heard keys jingling and dainty steps echoing across the marble entry, but the familiar sounds didn't ease his outrage. This time he wasn't about to listen to her groveling lies about her whereabouts. No, she needed to be punished. After all, aerobics classes never last three hours. He was sure she was up to no good again.

ᏬᎯᏫ

The call came in at 2:43 according to Eric's clock radio. The ringing jolted him from his restless sleep. He had been tossing, turning and dreaming about Amanda and the dilemma he found himself entwined in—not the ideal formula for a good night's sleep.

Eric, reached for his alarm and began to pound. He was groggy, with his heart beating a mile a minute. After continual attempts to silence it he realized the noise didn't cease and, in fact, was coming from his other bedside table. With his brain functioning just above oblivion, he rolled over, laughed at himself and reached for his ringing telephone.

"Hello," Eric muttered as he sat up with bloodshot eyes at half mast.

"Eric, is that you?" asked Nurse Clooney. The sound of that sweet old lady's voice was all too familiar. This time it was filled with worry.

"Yes," Eric answered. Her urgent tone made him fearful of bad news to come.

"I know this is none of my business, and I'm sure I'm breaking a few rules by calling but your 'sister' has just been admitted. She has been beaten, and is in serious condition."

He was too stunned to speak.

She continued, "Whoever did this to her should be locked up and they should throw-"

"I'll be there in 10 minutes. "

❧

It appeared as if they were stitching the cut on her head while they simultaneously iced and bandaged other areas. Amanda lay lifeless on a gurney in the emergency room, surrounded by a medical team that seemed to be proficient in patching her wounds. Her fair skin was illuminated by the intensity of the lights. Her eyes were closed and her face expressionless.

Nurse Clooney rounded the corner with two non-vending machine cups of coffee and a warm smile to soothe Eric's obvious fear.

"They'll be finished with her soon. She's stable and will be moved to a private room. Why don't we talk in the waiting room?" She gestured down the hall to the right and spilled a few drops of coffee in the process. "Oh, brought you some coffee. Hope it doesn't offend your dietary regime! I almost grabbed some donuts but I know you health nuts don't touch pastries with ten-foot poles!" They managed to smile and headed for the waiting room.

As they entered the vacated, stark room, Eric grew nauseated in its pungent 'sickly' smell.

"Before I tell you anything Eric, I need to know your relationship to Amanda Black. This 'sister' get-up isn't fooling me a bit." Nurse Clooney was more serious than he thought her capable. She looked directly into Eric's eyes, and the lines in her forehead grew deeper while her hand moved to grasp his. Eric felt like he was in third grade confessing to sticking a spit wad to Ginger Wiley's chair. He told all, including the marina meeting just hours ago.

She seemed to digest the story but looked a bit dazed. After a brief pause she spoke in monotones as if she had forgotten Eric was in the room and was instead reciting to the wall. "Well, now we know what triggered him. The question is whether or not she'll press charges this time." She turned to Eric. "I'm not supporting your behavior either. "

"Wait a minute...my turn to be enlightened," Eric pleaded. "This isn't the first time Amanda's been battered?" He paced around the room in horror. "She needs to file a police report and press charges."

"Maybe you'll give her the strength, but you'll have to be careful. Henry is a powerful man and his temper is—as you see—out of control." Nurse Clooney glanced at the clock. As the conversation came to a close, she slipped Eric her home number and assured him that he could call if he needed any help.

Before the door was shut Eric asked, "Why didn't you recognize Amanda the day of the Dipsea?"

"Amanda looks a whole lot different without blood and bruises."

There were twenty-seven listings of the name Black in the Marin County phone book, six of which were preceded by an H or an A. Looking closer at the six, one number stood out to Eric as the one he had dialed last night. The address was in Tiburon and with some familiarity with the exclusive Marin city, he guessed it to be located among the million dollar homes that were sprawled on the hillside that overlooked San Francisco

and the Golden Gate Bridge. From the hospital, Eric figured
it would take less than twenty minutes to reach Tiburon.
Reassured that Amanda was stabilized but unfortunately still
unconscious, he was on a mission.

As he drove on Highway 101, clearly over the speed limit,
he kept one eye on the rearview mirror for cops. Patrols were
sparse but not uncommon, even on a Wednesday at 4:00 A.M.
He felt relieved to be driving south without the usual bumper-
to-bumper traffic and obnoxious diesel fumes made by so many
of the Mercedes and Mac trucks that frequented the freeway
during peak traffic times.

Eric's thoughts moved to Henry and what Eric's intentions
were if a confrontation with Henry occurred. His blood
pressure most certainly was on the rise and his underarms were
soaked as he approached the address. Two homes were located
toward the dead end; in one, the lights were on. The address in
his hand matched the number handsomely engraved on a pillar
beside the wrought iron gate to the lighted home.

Parking below the driveway, Eric set the emergency brake
and curbed the wheels. He ran his hands through uncombed
hair and continued to search his recklessly running mind for
his next move. His eyes ventured to his right, then he heard a
loud rustling in the bushes and immediately after, a bright light
shown in his eyes. His unlocked door was thrown open by a
half-crazed older man yelling at the top of his lungs. His words
were slurred and the smell of alcohol escaped with his screams.

"Who the hell are you and what are you doing on my
property?" He staggered and caught himself just prior to
impact with his cobblestone driveway. This belligerent fool
looked ridiculous in his P. J.'s and was, in no way, a threat, Eric
thought.

"Are you Henry Black?"

"Henry Kessler—and you must be my wife's new toy. You
are the cause of this ordeal and Amanda—that bitch—paid the
price." He belched and ran towards Eric with arms flailing out
of control. Before he reached Eric, he tripped and fell to the

ground. Eric had no intention of peeling him off the ground or checking for damage.

Eric arrived back at the hospital by three-thirty to find that Amanda had regained consciousness and had been transferred to the third floor. Nurse Clooney was nowhere in sight. Her replacement, assuming he was the next of kin, skipped the third degree and directed him to room 326. Sporadically parked in the corridors and clustered near the nurses' station were carts and freestanding pieces of the latest medical equipment. The lights were dim and an eerie sense of calmness lingered. The smell of sickness was unavoidable. Eric took deep breaths in an attempt to compensate for his queasiness. With fear and guilt he entered the room alone.

Surprised and embarrassed, Amanda looked away momentarily. "Quite the role reversal tonight, Eric!" Amanda's pained face made it close to impossible to enunciate. Eric was amazed that she could find any humor in her predicament. He wanted to hold her, but under the circumstances lacked any decision-making skills, and instead collapsed in her bedside chair. He tried to speak but tears interrupted. Her hand reached for his and together they cried as they squeezed.

"I'm the reason for your battered body, Amanda," he managed after a long silence. "What can I do to help?"

"You're here...I already feel better. " A seriousness came over her face. "You'd be smart if you left now, Eric," she said under her breath as she closed her swollen, sad eyes. She didn't open them again until three hours later.

FIVE

The juvenile curtains of Amanda's youth were drawn to catch any daylight that diffused through the ruffled collaboration covering her windows. Three days had passed since her release from the hospital and Amanda lay listless, staring into the darkness of her childhood room. The anchor of depression had dragged her to unfamiliar depths and she lacked the strength to fight.

Between the threatening calls from Henry, including numerous hang-ups, Eric called daily out of concern and hope that Amanda would be up to talking. The disturbances were so frequent that Amanda's mother turned off the ringer in Amanda's room to ensure her daughter the tranquility the doctors had recommended.

Gabrielle Black had lived alone for over a decade. She had neglected to alter anything in her only child's room. The modest home, located in the San Rafael hills in middle Marin, sat on a hillside in the midst of an oak thicket. Her taste, though far from extravagant, held a certain elegance and class. Aesthetics had always been important to Gabrielle and she liked to take some credit in Amanda's success in the world of design.

Since her daughter's beating, Gabrielle's mind was far from home decor. Her intuition always told her of an evilness that lurked beneath the surface of Henry's polished facade. Never could she have imagined the monster that existed.

Amanda had been secretive and especially protective of her mother since her father left twenty-seven years ago. In their mutual abandonment Amanda always felt the need to protect her from further pain, at all costs. The cost this time was a high price to pay. As her physical wounds healed, the mental ones began to radiate. According to her physician, frequent outbursts with long periods of silence and no appetite were to be expected. So far, she displayed a textbook example of Post Traumatic Stress Syndrome.

On this third day of recuperation, Gabrielle felt the need to let some light into her daughter's fragile existence. For starters, she tied back the curtains and tilted the blinds a notch or two. Fresh clipped flowers from the garden arranged beautifully brought fragrance and life to Amanda's sullen mood. A crispy Caesar salad, laced with homemade croutons, was being attempted when the kitchen phone rang. It was Eric and this time Gabrielle felt her daughter was up to talking. "It's Eric, honey...do you want to take it?" She whispered and pointed to the silent phone on her bedside table.

Amanda picked up. Her expression became immediately more alert as she nodded and reached for the phone. "Hello Eric." Her voice was raspy and had obviously been temporarily out of commission.

"I've been worried sick about you Amanda. How are you?"

"I've seen better days. But I'm eating and total darkness isn't as comforting as it was yesterday. My mother is taking good care of me and I think I can get through this." Her voice quivered and tears began to stream down her cheeks.

"I'm here for you Amanda. What can I do to make you happy?" Eric's tears poured from his eyes.

"You just have." Amanda handed the phone back to her mother and Gabrielle spoke to Eric with continued reassurance. "If Amanda's feeling up to it tomorrow night, why don't you join us for dinner?" The hope and sincerity were clear in Gabrielle's soft-spoken voice.

As Amanda's strength grew, so did her attachment and love for Eric. Much of her time was spent with lawyers and accountants, dealing with the divorce and business options. Any remaining time was spent with Eric. Three weeks passed and she was back on her feet, struggling to hang on to her favorite clients, even with Henry's frequent attempts to sabotage her long established rapport. Walking away with fifty percent of the clientele and starting a business of her own seemed her best option. By the looks of things, Henry's drinking was affecting his work, and would soon cause his downfall.

Amanda and Eric went out to eat occasionally, but more often consolidated their 'virgin' cooking skills to create delicious concoctions. Amanda would often say, "The only prerequisite to any scrumptious meal is low-fat ingredients and creativity!" Eric would reply, "And then we can 'pig-out' on chocolate cream torte and still come out ahead!"

Much of the stress of their early months together were alleviated with these evening collaborations, mixed with brisk gallops through Marin hillsides and hidden trails on Mount Tamalpais. The secluded trails were endless and allowed Amanda and Eric to explore new paths together. Friendly competition with one another kept them on their toes and always made for better runs.

At the start of the holiday season Eric and Amanda were dining at Salute, a yuppie Italian restaurant in the heart of San Rafael that drew a crowd of upwardly mobile professionals, both daily and nightly. The food was authentic and superb. The wine selection contained varietals from wineries throughout Sonoma county. The atmosphere was always lively, and if a patron requested one in advance, a private booth was almost always available.

Divorce proceedings were coming along, and since they had nothing to hide, Eric asked to be seated in the open seating area. Amanda looked a bit surprised but found Eric's reassuring glance comforting.

The crisp white tablecloths, surrounded by brass and oak accents, were illuminated by the midday sun as Amanda and Eric followed the waiter to their table. Eric couldn't help but notice the countless heads that turned to get a closer look, as Amanda, oblivious to the adhering eyes, walked towards the table and sat gracefully in her chair.

"For some reason, I'm starved today," Amanda said as she accepted the menu from the waiter. She took a sip from her water then placed her napkin on her lap.

"I'm always hungry when we're together!" He raised his eyebrows and smiled as their eyes remained attached to one another.

A few minutes later the smooth Chardonnay calmed her nerves, but the weight of someone glaring from across the restaurant put a damper on complete relaxation. At first she avoided meeting the onlooker's eyes. She refused to 'give in' to her paranoia until her glass was empty and her curiosity was raging. Her face went white and expression pained. Eric turned to look over his shoulder to witness Henry walking toward their table.

"You can handle this," Eric said reassuringly as he clenched his teeth. Amanda's panic eased momentarily. As Henry neared, it was apparent to her that he had put on some weight. The circles under his eyes were dark and his face looked red and wrinkly.

"Ah.... look at the lovebirds now. So cute and cozy!" Henry's voice was a few decibels too loud with a hint of slurring around the edges, giving the patrons some lunchtime entertainment.

"Do you honestly feel it necessary to make a fool of yourself this afternoon?" Eric was proud of his comeback.

Henry rested his palms on the table and leaned toward Amanda. "What's up with you? Cat got your tongue?" The rotten stench of alcohol made it nearly impossible for Amanda to stay put. She stood to leave, her knees almost collapsing under her weight. Her hands visibly trembled and her speech froze.

"Are you afraid you might get some more of what you deserve, bitch?"

Eric called on every bit of his strength to stay in his seat and give Amanda an opportunity to stand up to the bastard. Henry suddenly raised his arm in Amanda's direction and the red line was crossed. Eric was on top as the punches began to impact in both directions. Glasses, silverware and table decor were thrown about as Henry and Eric rolled under the table, knocking it over in the process. Only minutes later, the sound of sirens were heard. Simultaneously the owner and three hundred pound cook peeled Eric from Henry. In the midst of the commotion, Amanda gathered herself and left the restaurant. The police entered in a flurry and witnesses were hovering and spouting their versions as the two opponents sat, still stunned at the explosive episode that had occurred.

Sergeant Arnoni made his way through the excited crowd, politely ignoring the witnesses who wanted a piece of the action. "Excuse me.... I'll be back for a statement after I talk to both parties involved...please step back...thank you..." He made his way to Eric, pulled up a chair beside him, slipped a pencil and a small yellow pad from his back pocket and began the brief interrogation.

"Okay, let's begin with your name and then I'd like to hear your interpretation of what took place this afternoon." Sergeant Arnoni was direct but not threatening and allowed Eric to calm down, gather his thoughts and speak clearly.

"Henry, the jerk who initiated the fight, is my girlfriend's ex-husband." Eric motioned Sergeant Arnoni in Henry's direction and continued his disclosure. "He has a history of physical abuse where my girlfriend is concerned, and I believe I came to her defense not a moment too soon. When he raised his arm in a threatening manner toward her face, after throwing a bunch of verbal threats at both of us, I lost it. I may have overreacted, but didn't want to gamble with the woman I love." It was at precisely this moment that Eric realized Amanda's absence. At first he was frantic but managed to hide his emotions. He mustered up a couple of reasons for her disappearance and probable destinations, which calmed his nerves slightly.

Within an hour and a half the excitement had died down, most of the patrons had gone back to work and the restaurant had been pieced back to its original beauty. Henry was slapped with a small sum to cover the broken glass and a table leg. He was also given a warning about his behavior by Salute's general manager. If he hadn't been such a longtime customer, he probably would have been forbidden to patronize the establishment for good.

Amanda almost didn't notice the steep slopes of Wolfe Grade as she neared her mother's home. Automatic pilot had moved her legs from the restaurant, down Fourth Street and up through the San Rafael foothills. She could think of nothing but getting away from the violence and finding solace in a quiet, safe environment. Her body felt numb, except for her bare feet, which were stinging with every step. Her pumps were tucked neatly in her purse with just the heels peeking out the top. Amanda's eyes were red and swollen and her hair was pulled back in a severe pony tail in order to keep it out of her face. Sweat beads had formed on the tip of her nose about two miles back and her soaked shirt was sticking to her back.

As the road went from pavement to gravel, the sound of the distant traffic began to decrease. The volume from the birds and other wildlife increased. At the sight of Gabrielle's house and the inviting wicker furniture on the front porch, Amanda began to come out of her daze. Behind her she heard a familiar hum. As she turned she met eyes with Eric. He slowly pulled the Saab beside her, unrolled the window and spoke as he reached his left hand toward her.

"I'm sorry you had to witness that, Amanda. I lost my temper. I wasn't about to let him touch you. Are you O.K.?"

Amanda, now in tears, held her head down, making it almost impossible for Eric to read her.

"I've been driving all over town looking for you. I don't want to lose you, Amanda." Eric's voice sounded tired and desperate.

"The walk was good. I'm a little shook up...I. . I had to leave. I hope you understand. I want that monster out of my life." Amanda walked toward the porch, eyes focused straight ahead, as she reached for Eric's reassuring hand. She turned and gazed into Eric's eyes only to notice that he too was crying.

Dusk came as Amanda and Eric embraced on the delicate wicker loveseat, Amanda's head resting silently on Eric's chest. No words were spoken. No words were needed.

SIX

One Year *Later*

Driving north on 101 for an hour put Eric, Amanda and Kelsey, their two-month-old yellow lab, in Guerneville. It was an unusually warm, dry, spring day and they intended to fill it with amusement on the Russian River.

Eric's intentions were far more complex. They included romance, a proposal and an engagement ring. The divorce was now final. In Eric's mind, the finale would come with Amanda's agreement to take his hand in marriage. He stopped at the small-town market, telling Amanda he needed a soda, but his plan was to pick up some chilled Kendall Jackson Chardonnay and some flowers. Amanda, putting in her order for some fresh juice walked Kelsey behind some overgrown bushes so the dog could relieve herself. Eric quickly hid the wine and irises in the hatchback, next to the picnic basket stuffed with cheeses, squaw bread, fruit and Toblerone chocolate.

The adventure began to peak after Eric rejected Amanda's suggestion to stop at the popular Johnson's Beach. Since her marriage to Henry, she had vowed to never let a man control her again. Sometimes her defensiveness was amplified by her past, which caused her to anger easily. Eric was struggling to hold back his smile and attempted to give a feasible reason for his refusal.

"There's a better spot up the road. More room for Kelsey and more private for us. You won't be inhibited when you decide to bask in the nude!" He said this with a straight face and his usual dry sense of humor. As he drove, he kept one arm on the wheel and with the other caressed her inner thigh.

"Oh, you're doing this for me and Kelsey," she teased and began to lighten up, realizing Eric was not trying to overpower her suggestion.

Stepping out of the car and overlooking the cliff and dense foliage, they were able to see the small private beach below. Still unsuspecting, Amanda threw on her backpack and forged ahead trying to keep up with Kelsey.

"This is gorgeous, Eric. I'll meet you down there. Hope the trail isn't infested with poison oak."

Eric grabbed the picnic basket, wine and flowers and placed them carefully inside his 'flea-market' blanket. He awkwardly felt for the small box containing the ring with his left hand as he hoisted the bundle down to the beach. With proposal material intact, he reached the beach and watched Amanda tossing a stick into the river and commanding Kelsey to 'fetch'. From Eric's perspective, laughter, praise and splashing were the predominant sounds, dominated only by his beating heart.

He carefully spread the blanket in the partial shade of an ancient redwood. Noticing that Amanda's back was to him, Eric quickly deposited the flowers, wine and small box behind a nearby bush. With that accomplished he sat on the blanket, wiped the newly formed sweat from his brow and began to relax. Deliberately falling to one side while reaching inside the basket for a soda left him lying on his side. The mild sunlight felt therapeutic as it penetrated his golden Norwegian skin. Kicking off his shoes and closing his heavy eyelids coincided with Kelsey's direct mount on Eric's entirety. With Kelsey's wet, sandy paws shivering with excitement and drooling tongue licking with love, all Eric could do was reciprocate.

"Time to get that lazy butt up now. We don't want you growing an 'accountant' body do we?" Amanda slipped her backpack from her diminutive shoulders, unzipped the main compartment and recovered a Frisbee. Tossing the pack on the now sandy and tousled blanket, she ran toward the river. "Go out for a pass, Eric."

Without thinking, he stood, ran full force ahead, but staggered over the wild heap that scampered between his legs. Kelsey let out a screeching yelp. Amanda turned toward the commotion and saw Eric trip over Kelsey and fall near a hollowed log. A putrid odor assaulted her nasal passages. Looking to her left, she caught a fleeting glimpse of a small black-and- white animal with tail erect.

Stunned, Amanda's face went white and her expression showed fear. Kelsey, apparently fine, began barking like a hound and chasing the skunk. Amanda's face changed as her uncontrollable laughter erupted. She managed a few words as she continued laughing, cross-legged now to stop herself from peeing her pants. Tears were streaming down her blushed cheeks as she held out her hand to help Eric to his feet.

"If you're trying to turn me on, I think you should try a different approach. "

"Say another word and I promise to rub my body all over yours." Eric could hardly stand his new 'scent' and began stripping and flinging his clothes as if performing a strip tease. With haste, he darted behind the bush, managing to grab the ring without stirring Amanda's curiosity. With a devious smile spanning the full width of her face, Amanda imitated Eric as she too stripped.

"Last one in the water is a rotten egg!," Eric yelled as he ran toward the river.

Tightly enclosed in his hand were the makings for the perfect moment.

Amanda, still cracking up over the incident, deliberately kept her distance as she trailed Eric, his aroma and naked buns. "I guess we'll both be rotten if I'm last," she managed between her giggles.

Moments later Kelsey returned and began swimming around their intermingled bodies. The tone had changed from playful to serious as they made love in the water. Amanda's back was arched and head thrown back in ecstasy, exposing her sensual breasts. Eric carefully held her body as he moved inside. Aware of nothing else, the two enjoyed each other's bodies and felt a connection neither had ever experienced with other lovers.

Kelsey decided to join the fun. Dog paddling toward, she scratched Eric's bare back, ending the passionate heat of the moment. Although Amanda longed for more, Eric couldn't stand the pain on his back.

"Oh, Kelsey, you stinky hound, you.... I think I'm gonna have to tie you to the hood of the car on the way home." He grabbed Kelsey and gave her a bear hug.

"Don't be so sure the stench is all emitting from her," Amanda interrupted as she withdrew from the interlude and walked up toward the blanket. The redwood and pine trees, laden with ferns and wild flowers, gave Amanda the sense of complete privacy as she shook and re-situated the worn blanket.

Eric approached their picnic area to find Amanda lying face down with a tattered straw hat shading her ivory-colored face. A bottle of sunscreen emblazened "Coppertone 45" sat by her side, causing Eric to momentarily shift his focus from her back side in its entirety.

"Never a moment's rest around here," Eric said sarcastically. "I guess you expect me to immerse your body in this lotion?" As he continued, he set down the ring, reached for the flowers and wine, fortunately still perky and chilled. "I just have one favor to ask of you, before I apply the sunscreen. "

"Yes?..."Amanda lazily replied.

"Will you marry me?"

Amanda hesitated while the question was transmitted and relayed to her brain. She rolled over to find Eric on his knee holding what appeared to be an engagement ring, a bouquet of flowers and a bottle of wine resting on his supporting leg. Amanda was in complete awe before the tears welled up and overflowed. She reached for him and was rewarded with a long embrace, topped with a passionate kiss of the highest caliber. Time seemed to stop as they held each other. Kelsey, now exhausted, curled up beside them, she seemed to sense their need for space and watched her masters with a hint of bewilderment.

"The only thing I didn't plan was to propose in the nude, but the added flair will definitely make this moment more memorable, don't you agree?" Eric said with a hopeful smile.

"Yes."

"Yes, you agree, or yes you'll marry me?"

Amanda leaned back from the embrace looked Eric directly in his eyes and uttered, "Both."

Eric stood as he held Amanda, screamed at the top of his lungs and twirled her in excitement.

SEVEN

The alarm was set to the most obnoxious 'RAP' station for the sole purpose of ensuring complete wake up. This morning was no exception. The 'Gangstas' were rapping at full throttle, jolting Eric from his quiet slumber. He sat up, pounded the 'off' button, glanced at his digital clock, which read 6:54, and realized the insanity of arising at this hour on a Sunday morning. He scrunched his pillow and fell back to sleep.

At 7:40 his doorbell rang and Eric immediately realized what he had done. A quick hand stroke through his tousled hair and straight to the door in his boxer shorts. Amanda reviewed the situation as soon as the door was ajar.

"Good thing I offered to drive this morning."

Eric was already sprinting back toward his bedroom, digging feverishly through a pile of questionably clean garments.

"Unlike you, Amanda, I have the capability of getting ready in under two minutes." He hopped on one foot as he put one leg then the other into his wrinkled running shorts.

Sure enough, they were heading for 'The Run to the Heavens' race in Eric's predicted time. Eric sported the 'wrinkled-grunge' look as he rubbed his tired eyes while Amanda sat silent and ready for a challenge in her color-coordinated warm-ups.

With the slight aroma of 'skunk' still lingering, even after Eric's attempts at the tomato bath and the half hour scrub with deodorant soap as well, Amanda remarked, "Your race strategy is obvious and, I might add, quite original! And don't pretend you can't smell yourself," she added with a smirk.

Eric burst into laughter to the point where his eyes were watering. "Well, you know what they say about body odor."

Amanda, now also laughing almost hysterically, added, "No, Eric, I flunked B.O. 101, please enlighten me!"

Eric crouched to lace his shoes, "People, myself obviously excluded, with chronic body odor are unable to recognized their own stench!"

"What have I gotten myself into," she added sarcastically.

Arriving at the race with thirty-five minutes to spare, Eric and Amanda had time to register, adjust and secure their bibs, and use the 'facilities' to drain the anticipation, recycled coffee and liquids. A quick stretch and jaunt through the private school grounds left them both warm with ample amounts of adrenaline flowing. The race director called the start and Eric and Amanda were off, along with five hundred other participants, all eager to reach the top and back to finish the steep, challenging six-mile scenic race.

The first half mile was flat, paved and competitive. Careful maneuvering was mandatory to keep from being tripped or stampeded. Resisting the games the mind can play at this point was always difficult for Amanda. Not only was she feeling winded, but many of the stronger runners began to pass her. Eric rubbed her arm gently as he forged ahead. "Good luck hon!" were the last words he spoke. Amanda knew she had set a good pace when she noticed only three women ahead.

The morning was foggy and cool with the sun beginning to break through near the peak of the mountain, three miles ahead. As she made the climb, the views began to expand in all directions. It was the only distraction from her exhaustion, and, when even the beauty wouldn't suffice, a man playing the bagpipes eased her pain tremendously. She felt a new exhilaration and grabbed a second wind and rode it out while she passed a woman with massive 'quads' and equally supportive calves. Sweat was oozing from every pore and her heart rate was sustained at its maximum until she reached the peak, now fully adorned in sunshine.

Eric was nowhere in sight and, most likely, hanging in the

lead pack of runners consisting of only elite athletes capable of holding their position in the front.

A few months ago Amanda, nursing a twisted ankle, had had the opportunity to witness Eric as he fought for a spot in the top ten at the Houlihan's to Houlihan's race. Nine men in addition to Eric were fighting for the best time. Nowhere had she witnessed such grace and strength, working in sync so beautifully. Eric ran with huge strides and determination and took an amazing second place, shaving off 45 seconds from his best time in previous years. Tears were streaming as she jumped for joy.

She felt proud as her love and admiration grew.

Another half mile was covered as Amanda continued to daydream. The downhill was smooth and the grade not too hazardous yet. She felt so incredibly light as she stayed at these flying speeds, conscious of only the breeze cooling and evaporating the sweat on her damp face. In the distance she began to hear the cheering from the crowd at the finish line. With approximately a mile to go Amanda snapped back into full consciousness. With that, came the pain in her legs and lungs. The last portion was rugged. Rocks were toppling, causing mini-avalanches as she fought to keep her footing. She approached the finish and could hear Eric cheering for her. Catching a glimpse of his shirtless physique and handsome face always gave her the power to sprint the last hundred yards. Her lungs felt like bursting as she fought to pass two contenders for a ribbon. She could hear nothing. Even her vision was intruded upon as her nausea rose. She used every muscle fiber and brain tissue to concentrate on picking up speed at this exhausting moment. To Amanda's surprise, her legs obeyed her brain and in the final fifty yards she passed both women.

Eric stood at the end of the chute, filtering the sometimes clumped finishers into a single file line, with open arms and lifted, twirled and embraced Amanda simultaneously. As soon as she caught her breath and replenished some fluids she said, "Did you have a good run?"

Eric, still energized from his fiance's victory, laughed.

"Does 'it sucked' give you any indication?" He led her toward an inviting grassy area, perfect for sprawling and relaxing. "Soon after passing you I noticed my shoe lace was untied. Why I forgot to double tie it is beyond me—and don't tell me it had anything to do with oversleeping," he said with a smile. "While struggling with the idea of finding a good time to tie it, watching my competition pass, I apparently stepped on the lace and landed head first on the fire trail." Eric displayed the scrapes on the palms of his hands, then pulled the hair off his forehead to uncover an almond-size goose-egg.

Smiling, with sympathy, Amanda said, "When are you going to control your male hormones, Eric? Running this hard can be hazardous to your health. You'll always be a 'stud' in my eyes, even if you don't win. Next time, tie your shoe right away, and forget the strategies.... Anyway, not everyone can win!"

EIGHT

Eleven Months *Later*

The old church was nestled on a San Anselmo hillside. The stained glass reflected brilliantly against the mahogany woodwork and ornate architecture. The high ceilings were adorned with colorful frescoes. Eric sensed his nervous anticipation rise as he waited in the groom's quarters with Mike. Everyone he'd ever cared about sat in the pews before him. Eric peeked through the curtain at the front of church. Faces on the right side were not so familiar, but he recognized all of them.

Amanda's college acquaintance was working hard on the keyboards, playing an array of instrumental pieces from the seventies and eighties. Amanda had been adamant about replacing the organ with the piano, claiming the organ's 'funeral' sounds gave her the goosebumps. Eric had shrugged and gone along with the idea, but at this moment he began to appreciate the difference the piano brought to the most precious day of his life.

Thank God for the bottle of champagne Mike brought to the church, specifically to be guzzled as they adjusted their cummerbunds. The buzz was pleasant and calmed Eric's anxious nerves as the time approached. The wait seemed like an eternity as the pews began to fill. Every few minutes Mike would peek into the church and give Eric, who paced in his quarters, an update on the new arrivals.

"A couple of matronly women with dyed red hair are being escorted to the left side...together...let's see,

I'd say conservatively four hundred pounds. I'll call them Aunt Hildegarde and Velma!" Eric burst into laughter but immediately caught himself as he worried he might be audible to the "spectators."

"Would you stop your wisecracks for one minute and fulfill your duties as my best man. I'm having trouble opening this bottle I brought...I know this is your specialty." Eric pulled the expensive bottle of Chardonnay from a red duffle sitting beside the vanity. He handed the bottle and opener to Mike as he fumbled some more in the duffle then recovered two carefully wrapped wine glasses.

Mike removed the cork as Eric unwrapped the antique glasses his grandmother had given him as a boy. Mike was anticipating some 'mush' and knew the moment was now upon him as Eric spoke.

"Mike, you've been my best friend for a long time and I want you to know how happy I am that you are my best man." Eric poured just enough for a toast. His eyes were glassy and his tone was more serious than usual.

"Well, I'm happy to be here and am looking forward to the day when you can do the same for me." It was a true rarity when Mike spoke without sarcasm.

"Do you think that is going to happen in this lifetime?" Eric gave Mike a pat on his back.

After making a toast to their friendship, they embraced and walked from the groom's quarters to an alley leading to the altar. Mike peeked around the corner to witness two beautiful girls, one of whom resembled Amanda, sitting in the second pew.

"Does Amanda have any sisters?"

"No, she's an only child. You're probably looking at her best friend Helen. They could pass for sisters, couldn't they?"

An all-too-familiar expression evolved on Mike's face.

"Don't worry," Eric said, "I won't forget to introduce you. Just don't get too drunk before your 'best man' speech. And by the way, can you keep it rated PG for the more innocent ears attending today?!"

The chauffeur slowed a bit as he turned onto Sir Frances Drake Boulevard to allow Amanda and Eric their moment of glory, waving out the sunroof of their rented Rolls. The day was sunny but the temperature mild for July.

The wedding had gone without a hitch, with one exception on Amanda's part. Toward the end of the ceremony, purely out of nervousness, Amanda started to leave the altar just as the pastor announced that the groom should kiss the bride. Laughter broke out, significantly reducing the nervous tension in the church. Fortunately, the ice was broken in the family's reception to follow. The photographer posed the bride and groom alone, and with various family members and best man and Sally, Amanda's Maid of Honor, as the others went on ahead.

"Trying to leave me at the altar, babe! Last minute second thoughts, eh?" Eric was playfully teasing as he nudged Amanda closer still, both waving to all the roadside commotion they were causing.

"Just playing hard to get...babe. " Amanda smirked and leaned closer yet as she laid a wet and juicy one right smack dab on his lips. Horns honked and onlookers screamed at the latest show of affection.

Mike, sucking up all the attention from below and still a bit high, was also enjoying the view of Amanda's sexy ankles. "I knew there were perks to being the 'best man', but I never imagined..." he said as he peeked up through the sunroof, eyebrows animated, for a reaction. "I know it hasn't stopped you in the past, but she's a married woman," Eric yelled from above, as he laid another 'wet' one on his new wife.

Amanda knew Mike's comments were harmless and decided to take part in his flirting game. "Come on guys, there's enough of me to go around. You are coming on the honeymoon aren't you, Mike?"

The driver, feeling he had eavesdropped on more than enough, pushed the power button and the inside window slowly rolled up as he turned into the Marin Arts and Garden Center for the reception. The manicured gardens were ideal for the day's festivities.

As the waiting guests caught a glimpse of the limo, a receiving line began to form. Eric helped Amanda down from her rooftop seat, and out of the limo. The bridesmaids and groomsmen and close family members were already busy with introductions.

The first person to greet the newlyweds was Mona Bixby. First Eric and then Amanda embraced her.

"Congratulations, you both look absolutely stunning," Mona said as she held their hands and gave them each a hearty squeeze.

"You look pretty stunning yourself," Eric added.

"Go on you two. I'll see you later." Tears filled her eyes as memories of her late husband came flooding in.

Eric and his bride took fewer than two steps before they were bombarded with the immediate family and friends on both sides. Tears, embraces and many congratulations came from all directions.

Nurse Clooney came up to them. She was adorned in a lavender suit with matching hat and shoes, which was becoming to her and quite an improvement over her usual white or pale green scrubs. "You have to admit I saw the spark from the beginning," she whispered in Amanda's ear.

Amanda smiled, "This is just like a romantic fairytale."

"Happily ever after from here on out, right?" They embraced and Amanda felt so secure in the soft fleshy breasts of her good friend. She turned to see Eric and her mother, Gabrielle, holding hands, both with joy flowing from their eyes.

"Mom, are we going to have to break into the second box of Kleenex?" Amanda said as she put her arm around Gabrielle.

"I wasn't expecting to be such an emotional wreck. It's just that I couldn't be happier for you." She reached for another tissue and blotted.

Champagne was circulating through the crowd as Eric and Amanda planted themselves at the end of the receiving line.

Mike zeroed in on the single women, metamorphosing into the perfect gentleman. Sally introduced herself then made a bee-line for the kitchen to make sure everything was running smooth.

Brick and Silvia were so proud of their son, Eric, and had begun the first of many toasts. Mitch and Kenny, Eric's older half brothers, although not close, both traveled great distances to attend their brother's big day. They both brought their growing families and many warm embraces.

"Baby 'bro' finally decided to tie the knot," Mitch said as he shook Eric's hand and simultaneously patted him on the back, as men do when they aren't quite comfortable with an embrace.

"Yes, and this is my beautiful bride, Amanda." Eric squeezed her hand as he complimented Amanda.

The stimulus of having every important person in both their lives, currently in their presence was almost too much at times. Introductions were constant and fortunately going pretty smoothly. Amanda was amazed at how well she handled Edward, her father, and his new wife. Amanda's childhood memories of her father prior to the divorce were sparse and practically nonexistent afterwards.

Amanda recalled not fitting into Edward's new life after he left. His new wife and two young stepchildren took center stage. To ease his guilt, he sent birthday and Christmas cards stuffed with exorbitant amounts of cash and empty promises of visits that never happened. The token unexpected phone call once or twice a year were the only other attempts at a relationship. At first the rejection was almost unbearable, and through the years Amanda's pain had grown into anger. Amanda knew that Henry was simply an attempt to replace the father she never had, and now it was clear why she withstood the abuse in her first marriage— fear of losing another father figure, even if it meant taking the abuse.

Standing before her was a man she didn't know, or care to know, for that matter. "Is that you, Edward? You've changed since your last photograph a few years back." She managed a cordial handshake and an unidentifiable grin towards the 'wicked stepmother' who surely had had a hand in Edward's negligence. Eric was by her side and was already reaching for Edward's hand just as any eager son-in-law would. After all, Eric was the one who convinced her to invite Edward. Briefly, Amanda neglected reality and pretended the moment wasn't flawed by the past. Watching her flesh-and-blood father and her husband shaking hands on her wedding day was like viewing a film in slow motion. Both so unbelievably handsome, with strong, broad shoulders and narrow athletic hips, so lean and masculine with chiseled faces. The kind that instead of sagging and shriveling, only improved with age. Firsthand evidence was visible on every square inch of her father's being. The flash ended and Amanda snapped out of her illusionary moment of bliss. She coaxed Eric to move along in the receiving line and moseyed towards the head table where the four-course dinner was to be served shortly.

As they neared the table Amanda began to feel the effects of the champagne tingling in her forearms. Extra giddiness was sounding in her voice, which was now turned up a decibel or two. She leaned closer to Eric and cupped her hand as she whispered into his ear, "Hey babe, do you think people would notice if we disappeared into the cloak room for a short rendezvous?"

Eric smiled, turned his mouth towards her ear and replied, "You had better stop talking like that unless you're ready for something really enormous to come forth." Eric subtly gestured towards his 'manlihood' as he pulled out a chair for his bride.

Amanda laughed out loud. "You had better watch your body language. I think the photographer caught that last gesture." She carefully scooted her chair toward the table.

Mike arrived at the table with two newly acquired escorts. "Eric, Amanda...do you suppose we could make room for these two beautiful women? I don't want to break any etiquette rules or get on your wrong side, Amanda!" Before he had finished his sentence, Amanda had given the O.K. nod. Eric pulled up two extra chairs.

"Just as long as we save this spot for Sally I don't mind a

bit," Amanda said as she squeezed the hands of her cousins who both seemed to be in the "running" for tonight's one night stand.

The harpist was playing a soothing piece when Sally joined the small gathering at the head table. Complete efficiency with an equal abundance of confidence and brains came striding along with the entire package. Her full lips enunciated with perfection as she spoke. "The first course is on its way and it looks absolutely beautiful. Almost too good to eat!" She smiled as she introduced herself to the cousins and continued, "Your Wedding Planner is really on top of things. "

"It's the perfect Wedding for the perfect couple." Mike chimed in, as the focus was diverted from Sally. "Let's propose a toast." He picked up his knife and began lightly tapping it against his fine crystal stemware. The high familiar pitch had the room down to a whisper in a matter of seconds. Mike stood, the room went silent and the guests were all ears.

"I've known Eric since third grade and we've been best friends ever since. He always seemed to have all the luck and Amanda is proof that he hasn't lost the touch! As a couple....... . " The toast went on for a few minutes as the room grew teary eyed at the touching ensemble Mike had prepared with such skill, making it seem that it was straight off the cuff.

As Mike sat he turned to not only shake Eric's hand but to make note of the impression his eloquent speech had upon both of Amanda's cousins. One quick glance and Mike knew he had his choice for the evening.

The wedding progressed through dinner, more toasts, and the first dance. The guests were having a ball as they observed the cake cutting and "bite exchange" carried out with the tenderness everyone expected. Amanda exposed her leg as Eric pulled the garter from her thigh to her calf and off her dainty foot. The striptease music was blaring to add to the moment. Eric turned his back to fling the garter towards the crowd of unmarried men and boys. The hoot and howls could be heard for miles, and when Mike caught the garter after risking injury when he hurled himself in the center of the group, pushing aside a few gentleman just before colliding with the floor, the volume increased at least three decibels. Mike, admitting that the garter was worth a bruise or two, took a bow and helped Amanda to a small stage to toss her bouquet.

As luck would have it Mike's new love interest caught the flowers and was playing into the palm of his hand the rest of the evening. Eric and Amanda could have continued the celebration all night long but were coaxed by Amanda's mother and Sally to get to their awaiting hotel suite at the top of Nob Hill. The guests were more than eager to give the bride and groom a heavy sprinkling of bird seed as they escorted the new couple to their car, now almost unrecognizable through the shaving cream, streamers and "Just Married" memorabilia plastered to the exterior.

After the slam of the car door, the only audible sound was that of the tin cans rattling as they bumped from their tied position on the rear bumper. Dusk was settling in as the sky began to turn darker shades of red and orange. Cars were sparse this evening on Highway 101, making the trip to the city all the more relaxing.

"Can you believe we're married, Eric?" Amanda was turned toward the back seat rummaging through some wedding paraphernalia apparently looking for something. "Yes, but I'm still in a daze.... the most wonderful dream.... pinch me occasionally Amanda. What are you looking for back there?" Amanda reached for Eric's right hand and gave it a big squeeze with her back still facing the dashboard.

"You can count on more than just a pinch when we get to the City, but right now I'm trying to uncover that bag of Doritos Mike left in here after the bachelor party! I'm starving. Something about being photographed while chewing takes away my appetite. I see it didn't hinder you a bit. Aaahah.... Here they are." Eric accepted the squeeze and took it farther as he caressed her shoulder and neck.

"My honeymoon night, and my bride will have Dorito breath! I think Ann Lander's will have to be informed." Amanda laughed so hard and unexpectedly that she accidentally catapulted a cheesy morsel which adhered itself to his cheek.

"And now you are spitting chunks on me! I wonder if Ann's got an emergency fax number!.... Would you please stop hogging and allow me a small handful?"

NINE

Three Months *Later*

The fall showers were welcome after five drought-ridden years. The vibrating sound of the lightest trickle was amplified by the skylight in the ceiling of their newly purchased condo. With tax extensions due at mid-month, Eric, like most CPAs, was inundated with work and had been putting in long hours at the office.

Amanda, alone and snug with massive pillows, nuzzled down farther into the covers as she turned the pages of the latest project she was compiling for a client. The soft sound of Phil Collins competed only slightly with the rain. Together the two sounds made beautiful harmony.

Amanda, with the help of Gabrielle, had decorated the room in a simple understated fashion. Creams and whites dominated, with an occasional splash of the most wonderful shades of green. The brass and iron bed had been Gabrielle's wedding present and was situated at an angle with a mature Ficus plant behind the headboard, where it was growing and thriving.

An abundance of natural light adorned the cozy master bedroom by day and the alluring twilight entered through the skylight by night. The rest of this two-bedroom charmer was nice, but Amanda spent most of her waking and of course sleeping hours in this favorite of rooms.

For a moment she paused from her work, rubbed her eyes, and wondered why she felt so tired. But she quickly remembered that her run had been longer this morning. She laughed out loud, realizing her physical sensitivities now that she was approaching her mid-thirties. Ten years ago, an extra couple miles would have made no difference.

Eric entered the condo at ten after ten to find Amanda lying on her notebook with pencil still in hand. How he adored her every characteristic: her full rosy red lips and long lashes and delicate facial structure. She was most beautiful when she slept, he thought. Eric shucked off his wrinkled clothes, clicked off the light and climbed into bed with his wife.

Amanda's eyes opened for the first time when he attempted to slide the notebook from under her head. A sleepy smile enriched her moonlit face. "What time is it, Eric?" She put her notebook on the antique bedside table and reached to pull herself closer to him.

"Time to make love to my wife and to satisfy her every need and desire...oh, and the clock says a little after ten. " Eric began unsnapping the negligee as she willingly complied.

Eric's eyes opened. With a slight twist of his neck he was able to make out the digital numbers on the face of his clock radio, which was next to the Ficus, on the bedside table. Amanda claimed that the clock was far from "aesthetically pleasing" and therefore needed to be camouflaged behind the branches. Six twenty-two, just eight minutes before the "rap" station would blare. As he reached for the off button, Amanda stirred and mumbled, but went right back to sleep.

Eric slid out of bed, walked straight for the master bathroom where he threw on his robe and peed simultaneously. Hoping that Amanda wouldn't misconstrue not flushing as careless and vulgar, he considerately left the dark bathroom to turn up the furnace and ground some fresh coffee beans. With that accomplished, he showered.

When he was finished he fully expected to see Amanda propped on her pillows, enjoying her coffee and ready to fire voyeuristic comments at him. Instead, she continued her deep slumber. She looked almost angelic with her face relaxed and partially exposed in the midst of sunken fluff. Her hair looked as if she had run a brush through it, laid down and hadn't moved a muscle. Eric was always amazed at her untousled beauty as she slept. After a few minutes of staring in awe, he decided to write her a love note instead of waking her from her peaceful slumber.

Amanda,
Hey sleepy-head, just couldn't resist watching
you sleep and couldn't muster the strength to
wake you from your dreams. I hope I didn't cause
you to be late to work, but if so I will surely
think of a way to repay you. Thank you for last
night. I look forward to all the nights we will
share in the future. I'll be late again tonight and
hope we can meet for lunch.
Call me
love Eric

Amanda woke with a start. She did a double-take when she looked up to the half-hidden clock, which read eight seventeen. Still disoriented, Amanda sat up and turned to see a cup of coffee on her bedside table. A smile came over her lips as she reached for the cup's handle only to find it and the cup itself to be room temperature. It was then that she noticed the note that had been placed with care, its corner tucked under the saucer to keep it from blowing to the floor.

As she read the note she felt like a schoolgirl whose heart skipped a beat upon receiving such a personal thought from a boyfriend. She brought the note up to her nose hoping to catch the familiar scent that she adored so.

Realizing how behind she was, Amanda sprung from her bed, made a beeline for the shower and was dressed and at her office in a matter of minutes.

As Amanda dove into the world of design, color, and dimension, her mind drifted to Eric. Before she knew it, her hand had pressed automatic dial and Eric's office line was ringing.

ᴄᴀ⊃

Eric was seriously beginning to wonder if he would get anything accomplished on this busy October morning. The phones had been ringing relentlessly since seven. Tina arrived at eight and was able to screen or temporarily satisfy some clients, lightening the flow considerably, but with two-minute intervals between rings, the day was looking bleak.

The familiar high-pitched clicking of high-heeled shoes echoed down the hallway, drowning out the low hum of the dueling Laserjet printers. Tina appeared at the threshold, toting a fresh pot of coffee and a stack of messages.

"Good morning Eric. Amanda is on line two. Do you have time to take it, or should I tell her you'll get back to her?" She entered the quaint cluttered office in search of his empty coffee cup. She found it sitting precariously on the slanted top of his computer monitor.

"Good morning Tina. I'll take it and thanks for all the screening...coffee too." Eric reached past some scattered files and picked up the receiver.

"Hi, sleepy head," he said as he picked up his freshly brewed Colombian.

"You were so sweet to leave me coffee and a love note. Promise me you'll never change?" Amanda looked up from her work and gazed at a watercolor print hanging on her wall.

"It's a guarantee." He turned in his swivel chair to grab a view of Mount Tam.

"Can I entice you to some lunch?" Amanda smiled as she doodled on the pad beside her phone.

"Sure, where do you want to meet?"

"I have a client to meet in Novato at eleven-thirty, so let's say one o'clock. Twelve-thirty if you're willing to make the trek up this way?" Her stomach growled and her head felt light. She hoped Eric would make it the earlier time in Novato.

"Mona has been raving about the 'Cacti' ever since it

opened. I'll just have to put in some extra time tonight. See you at twelve-thirty." Eric hung up and dove back into his never-ending files.

❦

Thank God for the Marin Bagel Company, Amanda thought as she headed North, sinking her teeth into the fresh warm grain. Just a small detour in central San Rafael had lead her to the long-established bagel factory. Pulling in to an almost unheard-of front-row parking spot reinforced the fact that her errand was well worth the effort. As she reached for her second and final pre-lunch snack, she began to feel less starving and definitely more alert.

She arrived at Bel Marin Keys as she swallowed the last bite of her second bagel. She pulled into the complex on Commercial Boulevard, put her car in park, tilted the rear view mirror to check her teeth for poppy seeds and quickly reapplied a new layer of apricot lipstick.

The office's facade was average, but upon entering the building she realized that a careful visual eye had aided her work on the beginnings of its' interior.

Selna Dewitt, office manager and vice president of Dewitt and Son's Contracting, looked older than her husband, John, by at least a decade. After meeting their four rather callous children she bore, Amanda attributed the premature pruning of her face to giving birth to, then attempting to de-barbarianize the young lads. Every attribute they possessed was as far from refined as one could stretch. Tobacco chewing, unshaven faces and foul mouths countered Selna's refined manners and graciousness.

Amanda had gathered this information in her one and only appointment last month with Selna, shortly after the build-out of the office had begun.

"Hi, Amanda...come, sit down. I have some fresh baked cookies and some tea." Selna motioned her toward the front office which was situated like a fishbowl between the outside and interior office spaces. "Your idea about the abundance of glass in my office...How can I thank you enough?"

"I don't deserve all the credit Selna. You need to think of me as a guide only. Your input and ideas have been splendid, which is more than I can say for the majority of my clients." Amanda sat politely at the temporary card table and took a Snicker-Doodle from the Lenox plate as Selna dipped tea bags and poured hot water from what appeared to be an antique pewter teapot. It was amazing to Amanda that in the midst of a build-out, Selna's obvious refinements still managed to surface.

"Well, we are at the final stages, which means, that for you, the fun has just begun." Selna shifted in her seat as Amanda pulled the various swatches and samples from her oversized leather briefcase.

"I've been dreaming of blues and mauves and since John has given me the go ahead to pick and choose as I like, I think it's settled," Selna said with finality and confidence.

"We'll simply have to narrow it down to a definite shade. And you were interested in wallpaper at our last meeting?" Amanda shuffled through a book full of various wall coverings. "I've placed bookmarks in the few I thought you might like. Each pattern comes in almost every color under the rainbow, so don't let the color throw you." Amanda leaned in closer to point out the particular wallcovering she was referring to.

Selna's eyes lit up as soon as the page was turned. "Do you mean to tell me that this beautiful landscape design can be made up in blues and mauves?"

Amanda's head tilted as the inquiry registered. "I can't say I've come across this request in the past, but I really think it will work. I'm sure the manufacturer won't have a problem with the dye lots."

"It's settled then. The paint I will leave up to you. I think this blue-gray carpet with the mauve borders will look great with all the furnishings we chose, don't you?" Selna looked so excited as she pointed to the carpet sample lying on the card table.

TEN

The iced tea seemed to fill in the cracks which were meshed with an abundance of bagels and cookies. An equal blend of corn and squaw bread, whole fresh beans and a variety of spices made for a magnificent aroma. The restaurant was packed, but Amanda's luck held. She was placed in a semi-private booth in a less chaotic corner. Full satiety was reached upon Eric's arrival at twelve thirty.

"Am I late?" Eric glanced at his watch as he leaned over to place a quick peck on her cheek.

"No, I'm early. My appointment didn't take as long as I intended. I've been here about fifteen minutes." She reached for her iced tea just as the waiter, clad in a jalapeño pepper shirt, began refilling her near empty glass. "Thank you," Amanda said.

The waiter turned, placed the pitcher on the buffet behind him and proceeded to describe the specials. They both half listened. Their appetite for food was dwindling as their appetite for each other grew.

Eric said, in one of his more professional voices, "I think we need just a few more minutes."

It was as if they could read one another's minds. Their laughter was muffled but not inaudible.

"How does a lunchtime rendezvous sound?" His left eyebrow undulated as he inquired.

Amanda's eyes lit up. "My car is stocked with fresh bagels."

"Bagels.... O.K., it's settled then. You slip out the back—

meet you at your car in two minutes." He pulled out his wallet, placed a five on the table.

They laughed all the way down Grant Avenue as Eric took the wheel in one hand and a bagel in the other. With no destination in mind they headed toward Novato Boulevard which eventually led to the backroads of Marin. "I guess I'll have to wing it when Mona calls for my review on the Cacti," Eric said with a chuckle. "Not necessarily, Eric. Don't forget I was there a full twenty minutes. The iced tea was great, along with the service and atmosphere!" Amanda reached over and slowly untucked Eric's shirt.

"You have a point." Eric drove slowly past Stafford Lake. I'll be in the clear as long as she doesn't ask about the entrees."

Amanda caressed Eric's face, neck and shoulders as he drove in an erotically heightened state. As soon as her hand traveled under his shirt, skin to skin, the heat had risen to the point of needing to either pull over or abstain from fondling completely. It was too late for option number two. Eric managed to find a somewhat secluded dirt road which seemed to lead to nowhere. He pulled over, put it in park and enjoyed the spontaneous passion.

Eric realized he would probably have to work through the night to make up for lost time today.

It was completely worth it, he thought.

The Cheese Factory, although a stone's throw from the city of Novato, gave one the illusion of being in the boondocks. The inescapable aroma of ripening cheese was evident as soon as Eric got out of the car.

"Whoa, maybe we should skip the cream cheese. If it gets any more pungent inside, I think I'd puke!" He sat back into the driver's seat and pondered the idea of plain bagels.

Amanda opened the passenger door, stepped out and took a vigorous inhale. "Ah...it brings me back to the time we came here for Miss Montgomery's fourth grade picnic. "Most of the kids were gagging at the stench. For some odd reason, it didn't bother me, and, in fact, by the end of the field trip, the smell had changed to a pleasant one." Amanda walked around to the driver's side to coax Eric from his hiding place. "Richard Holmes was the only boy...'man' enough, to look past the over-exaggerated gags and actually learn the process of cheese making. Come on, Eric. Prove to me you can 'hang' with it too."

"If Dick can handle it, so can I." He shut the door with a shove from his gluteals and reluctantly ambled toward the 'stinky' destination, one hand holding his nose, and the other, two poppyseed bagels.

The cow bells on the old wooden door sounded, alerting the elderly couple who ran the place. The woman came up from the back room wearing a white apron and hat. At best she stood five feet high. She was edging toward her seventies and sported an enormous gray braid that hung past her waist. She greeted the young lovers with a smile that exposed a few missing teeth.

"Hi, my name is Mabel, but most folks know me as Tiny. "

"Hi, Tiny, nice to meet you." Amanda recognized Mabel from the fieldtrip. She had thought she was ancient two decades ago! It was amazing the woman was still alive.

"Are you here for a tour, or just stopping through for a sample this afternoon? You know we've got the finest cheese in California." "We'd love a tour, if you have the time," Amanda chimed in before Eric had time to squirm his way out of the situation. Amanda elbowed him and gave him a quick smirk.

"Can you recommend a soft cheese for the bagels we brought?" Eric hesitantly raised the bagels and was praying she wouldn't suggest something too 'smelly.'

"With those poppyseed bagels, there's nothing better than aged Camembert." She was unwrapping a large cheese round when her husband joined them.

"Hand me them bagels and I'll fix you right up." He was closer to eighty and as sweet as could be.

"This here is my husband, Jim." Tiny, all smiles, was proud to introduce him.

Jim turned to his lovely wife as he continued to slather

the bagels in the Camembert. "I could use some help stirring the breakfast cheese when you get a minute. I'm sure this nice fellow," motioning to Eric, "wouldn't mind a bit. "

"Love to." Eric followed Jim and his two cheese-topped bagels in the back where the aroma grew with every step.

Jim's short stature dominated Tiny's by less than six inches. His white hair and sparkling green eyes surrounded by lines, complemented Tiny's features.

Amanda followed them and was in awe as they stopped in a room filled with stacked cheese rounds and two enormous vats of milk waiting its turn to become cheese.

ELEVEN

Thirty-five Years *Earlier*

The rickety stroller in which they were placed was filthy but served the purpose of transport, far better than lugging them from ride to ride at Walt Disney's dream land. Thankfully the day was overcast which helped with tolerance levels in the mazes, referred to as lines, on this Saturday afternoon. Remnants of pink cotton candy were clearly visible on the faces and hands of both young boys, who at the moment were mesmerized by Minnie Mouse and her acrobatic act. At the conclusion of the act, Minnie innocently reached down to pat the boys on their heads. The older one screamed, jumped from the stroller and ran the short distance to his mother. The father moved in closer to apologize and to come to the aid of his youngest, whose stroller was teetering as he attempted his own grand escape. A slow-motion camera seemed to roll as the helpless father watched his son fall. There was a loud thud, with a rush of blood as the child's head met the newly asphalted ground.

The terrified father scooped him up, grabbed a blanket from the stroller, then quickly applied pressure. He scrambled to catch eyes with his wife, who was motioning him toward a building with the Red Cross emblem posted in bold red paint. Briskly, but with extreme caution, he ran the hundred yards, thinking how lucky they were to be so close to medical assistance.

Only two teenage boys sat in the corner of the cramped

waiting room. One was having trouble breathing and was being assisted with an inhaler. An overweight medical assistant clothed in white, complete with cardboard nurses hat, greeted Mr. and Mrs. Edwards.

"Please, follow me; don't stop the pressure. The doctor is in the back with another patient. "

They hurried into the brightly lit hallway. Where it dead-ended, two exam rooms were located across the hall from one another. Room A was shut, but the screams that sounded from that direction were loud enough to temporarily drown out even Mitch's wails. The assistant motioned for the Edwardses to occupy room B as she lightly knocked on the adjacent room, and returned with the doctor in less than a minute.

"What seems to be the problem here?" the doctor asked. He glanced at the still- howling child and walked to the corner to bathe his hands in the porcelain basin.

"He fell from the stroller on the pavement right out front," Brick responded as the doctor peeled back the blanket to uncover the wound.

"It all happened so fast. Is he going to be all right?" Mrs. Edwards asked. The child began to calm down and the sobs decreased considerably.

"After three or four stitches he'll be as good as new. The bleeding has just about stopped. Will you continue pressure while I get the suturing supplies and check on my other patient?" The doctor moved with efficiency and skill, assuring the Edwardses that their baby was in good hands. He exited the exam room, putting Brick in charge of his younger child. It was then that Brick's color returned to his face. He wiped his brow and looked to his wife who managed a smile and attempted to start a conversation as she held Kenny, the squirming toddler in her arms.

"I know we've talked in circles in the past. I think it's time we faced reality regarding the third child that you feel will make our family complete." She paused, pushed the overgrown bangs from her face and continued with her head tilted somewhere between the floor and Kenny, who had started to emulate the breast stroke on the polished linoleum. "Today is the perfect example of what can happen when we are both here to protect the children. Can you imagine how it is when you're out on the road for weeks? They are more than a handful. Another child... for me is unthinkable." She looked Brick square in the eyes as tears welled up in hers.

Brick raised his gentle hand and gestured for her to come closer for a squeeze. She stepped forward with relief and was encompassed by her husband. In the past this topic had been met with controversy and argument. Only now had Brick changed his attitude.

The embrace she gave him was empty on her part. Brick reciprocated with a one-handed cuddle, as he continued to apply pressure to the baby's wound.

The doctor strode in with suturing materials in tote. He laid the tools gently on a sterile steel tray then checked on the wound. "It's done bleeding. I'll need you, Mr. Edwards, to hold his arms. I'll take care of the little tike's legs."

Gail Edwards thought this to be the perfect time to chase Kenny up and down the halls, since the thought of watching the doctor poke holes in her baby was enough to make her nauseated.

"Kenny, let's see how we can do the wheelbarrow in the hallway." Without the slightest arm-twisting, Kenny flew out the door and knelt down in the center of the hallway.

"Mommy, I'm ready for my first load. "
She grabbed his legs and they were off.

"It's O.K. honey, daddy's here." Brick firmly held Mitchell's arms as the doctor administered a mild anesthesia to dull the forthcoming pain. The baby had begun to scream and struggle, but within a minute, he calmed down and seemed oblivious to the suturing taking place on his head.

"That should do it, six stitches. Ten days to two weeks; these should be removed. Your pediatrician or you can do it, if you feel comfortable." The doctor bandaged the area, then turned to wash his hands. The assistant knocked on the door and then opened it, exposing only her cherub-cheeked face.

"Another patient has been placed in Room A—nosebleed."

The doctor replied, "I'll be right there." He shook Brick's hand, patted baby Mitchell gently, waved good-bye to Gail Edwards and was on his way.

A line for the monorail was forming a hundred yards from the Red Cross building. Briskly they walked; the baby in Brick's arms and Gail pushing Kenny in the stroller.

Brick had insisted on staying at the Disneyland Hotel for its convenience and ease with the two young children. Gail Edwards knew these were plausible reasons for choosing an expensive hotel, but realized the hidden agenda as well. She imagined the bragging at the numerous truckstops along his route. She found herself practically feeling sorry for the unfortunate coworkers who innocently struck up a conversation with Brick.

"Hard to get back into the grind after all that luxury, Bob. Just took the boys and the little woman to Disneyland. Ever stayed at the Disneyland Hotel? They sure know how to treat you with style. We're thinking of Hawaii next year, what about you?"

The scenario replayed several times when she realized the monorail had not only come to a halt, but Brick had exited with a child under each arm.

"Are you up to your daydreaming again, Sweets?" The familiar tone in Brick's voice jolted her from her trance and made her skin crawl. She instantly came up with her pat answer: "Here I am drifting when I should be paying attention." So far the reply had sufficed, but she suspected some curiosity or possibly worry on Brick's part.

The wind blowing softly in her face and the monorail's motion had soothed her discontent but in no way could repair the problems in their marriage. At times she wondered how Brick couldn't see her emptiness.

TWELVE

Eleven Months *Later*

The pressure was almost more than he could bear. On the one hand, there was Gabrielle who had jumped the gun, picking out a china pattern and planning a storybook wedding; and on the other were his parents, generous with what little they could spare for the sake of their son and his high hopes of completing his Pre-Med Bachelor's degree. His classes demanded one hundred and fifty percent. So far he had been able to stay afloat even with the abundance of outside interference thrown his way.

Last night's news had left him off balance, to say the least. He felt trapped in a world he had no control over. How would he manage with a baby, especially now when the financial picture looked so bleak.

Gabrielle was not a student. For the past three years she had been, thankfully, employed with the university administration offices. The job's earnings were meager but steady and would definitely help with the majority of the bills. It was all happening too fast. The doctor indicated she was beginning her eighth week. Soon her belly would tell all, and the profound protrusion would be a child he felt unprepared to father. Fear began to overwhelm his thoughts, and denial was his only ally and coping mechanism. The encircling light fixture above the bed pulled him further from reality and aided his hypnotic state. The longer he stared into the blur above him, the easier it was to pull away from the stress of reality.

The toilet had flushed innumerable times in a span of less than twenty minutes, finally breaking his semi-trance. He pulled himself from beneath the fluffy bedspread and knocked lightly on the bathroom door.

"Gaby,...are you O. K?" His severely wrinkled boxer shorts rode cockeyed on his hips with the flap open, exposing the skin to the right of his genitals. Feeling the odd draft, he straightened the shorts and listened for a reply.

"Let's just say, I know it's not the flu. Obstetricians across the country refer to it as morning sickness. Pregnant women should put some serious thought into renaming the 'ailment.' All- day sickness would be much more fitting! Oh God, here it comes again!"

He opened the door to witness his young, unprepared girlfriend of less than a year, retching and gasping for air, all the while never letting up on her grasp around the porcelain God. He came closer and held back her hair as he stoked her pale face.

"If it's any consolation, I read in medical text that you should feel better in a month or two. "

Gabrielle looked up as she flushed. He noted that her face sported a hue of green. She had dark circles under her tired eyes.

"You sure know how to make a girl feel good. I'll believe it when and if the time comes." She laughed and continued. "If you really want to help, Edward, why don't you make a grocery run today. The doctor informed me that nausea can sometimes be subsided with Saltine crackers. If you see any frozen French fries, please pick them up too."

Realizing there was less than two dollars sitting in his checking account and five days until his parents would be depositing their meager contribution, he attempted a reassuring expression while he responded to Gabrielle.

"Consider it done. They are going to have to restock the Saltines when I'm through!" He stopped the caressing just long enough to pull down a towel from above, fold it and pillow it under her weary head.

"What would I do without you, Edward?" She rested gently on her pillow. Her expression changed from apathy to bewilderment as she again spoke. "There's something I need to tell you." She paused as she lifted her head and turned to meet his eyes. "I know how much stress you've had to withstand, with school and all your financial worries...and now a baby. I haven't had the heart to tell you what happened at work."

Her tears crested then streamed down her delicate face. She pulled a tissue from under her sleeve, blotted her wet face and gathered her thoughts.

"Since your classes start early and frequently go into the evenings you haven't been aware of how long I've been ill. Sometimes I'm able to make it to work but, in the last month, I've spent many days camped out on the tile floor." She gestured toward the toilet, eyes affixed on the floor as her confession continued. Looking a little less ashamed, she managed to lock eyes with Edward. "I was only trying to spare you the worry. . I, . I know you're under a lot of pressure..." She took a deep breath. "To make a long story short, on the days that I did make it to work, my supervisors took note of my frequent trips to the bathroom and the lack of time spent at my desk. I knew they were getting fed up with me so I finally divulged our predicament to them. Instead of being understanding, they fired me."

The room went silent. Edward sat down next to his pregnant girlfriend, his back turned, and wondered how on earth they would manage. His dreams of becoming a doctor were shattering before his eyes as anger began to dictate his reactions. For the first time, terminating the pregnancy or putting the baby up for adoption came to mind as viable options. Edward was almost as surprised as Gabrielle to hear the crude words spewing forth from his mouth without rehearsal.

"If you would have been more careful we wouldn't find ourselves in a predicament like this now would we? Maybe we should look into other options for the baby. "

Gabrielle, feeling his apparent resentment like a blow to her heart, began to realize the shaky ground in which her vows would one day be resting. Resting...that is, if Edward went through with the proposal made only last night.

Propping herself to the erect position, she spoke with a mother's conviction. "With, or without you, I plan to raise this baby. Go ahead and leave...you're free...Neither I, nor this baby, have any intentions of screwing up your life." Her eyes began to tear and Edward could see slight tremors in her neck, but she continued to sit tall and brave.

Almost immediately, Edward wished he could retract his hurtful words. Completely confused in his anger and guilt, he exited the bedroom, walked through the narrow hallway which led him toward the front door. There he lifted his bomber jacket from the peg on which it hung and pulled his keys from a wicker basket placed on a desk below.

"I'm sorry, Gabrielle." He raised his voice enough to be audible to Gabrielle, not loud enough to arouse the busy-body neighbors. He opened the door and was on his way to no particular destination.

Circling the apartment complex on foot three times, the scenario of his life continued playing round and round with different conclusions attached to each path chosen. Getting nowhere fast, he changed his route and headed for the 7-Eleven, hoping a caffeine boost would lift his spirits.

Unsure of what he might find in his bedroom, he reentered his apartment and moseyed his way down the hallway to find Gabrielle sleeping like a baby in the midst of his bed. He sat on the bed Indian style with coffee cup in hand, sipping, staring and contemplating.

He reached down to stroke her blotchy face. She opened her swollen eyes, and at that moment he realized that he could never abandon his child. He would marry Gabrielle and give the child his name. For him, this marriage was based in principle rather than love. Somehow he would find a way. They would find a way.

THIRTEEN

Three Years *Later*

Edward had hit the snooze button numerous times, but each time he had delved right back into REM, where his recurring nightmare awaited him. The limbs of the still- screaming woman were completely severed. Blood was squirting in all directions and the scalpel was being handed like a hot potato from one medical student to another until it was forced into his trembling hand. He couldn't open his fist to continue the hand-off. A line etched on the poor woman's neck dictated the next cut. His hands suddenly felt like lead as his classmates stood watching. In the background, out of focus, but definitely taking note, was Professor Jacobsen. Determined not to fail, Edward began the incision. He attempted to focus on the neck, but for some reason his eyes were pulled toward the face. In his terror, he is met by his mother's eyes.

The ringing alarm saved him from the fright. This time he not only opened his eyes, but bolted from his bed. He picked up his ancient clock and kissed it numerous times.

Plagued with nightmares from the start, the entire semester was draining, both physically and mentally. He was beginning to worry if he could handle the Anatomy class and its continual dissections of the human body. Working the late shift at the local Mexican restaurant wasn't helping matters either. Between classes, work, and studying, sleep was always neglected. Now, with the nightmares, he felt his conscious hours slipping into a blur.

His student loans were escalating. Since his parents were

tapped out at the end of undergraduate school, he had been on his own for the past five years. With a little girl to support and no rich uncles, he had to work. He closed his eyes as he stood in the shower, hoping to somehow accumulate some quality rest before heading to class. Once again, he would be late to Advanced Cardiac Studies.

Dried, dressed, with instant coffee ingested, he was on his way. Spring time had always been his favorite time of year. He had limited time to enjoy its pleasures, but he made sure to take in the sights between classes. The flowering plum trees that lined the perimeter of Stanford's prestigious campus were in full, fragrant bloom. The grassy areas were especially green. The women had left their bulky sweaters behind and instead were clothed in lightweight dresses that looked translucent when backlit by the sun, giving life to the soft lines of their female bodies.

Edward's pace was quick and directed in an attempt to be less late. As he walked up the steps toward the building where his class was already in progress, a bright orange flyer caught his eye and pulled him closer for a better look. The flyer read:

—ATTENTION MED STUDENTS—
SPERM DONORS NEEDED
quick cash-completely confidential
for more information call:
Stanford Fertility Clinic.
332-2714

His face flushed as he looked first to his right, then over his left shoulder, making sure the coast was clear. Pretending to be interested in an adjacent flyer, he let two women in their translucent dresses pass before he tore a detachable phone number from the flyer. Stuffing the scrap into his backpack he continued on his way.

"Glad you could join us once again, Mr. Black!" The professor diverted his attention only to make the comment, then directed the class back to the image of coronary vessels on the overhead.

Finding a seat in the dark had become routine for Edward this semester. The front row was usually his best bet, and today was the only option available. Attempting to keep his disruption to a minimum, he quietly scrambled for a pencil and appropriate notebook.

His mind drifted momentarily to Amanda, his three-year-old who lived with her mother Gabrielle. The divorce had been especially difficult for her, and one day he hoped to make amends. For now keeping his head above water and his grades from slipping were his only concerns.

The student center was the popular hangout for the frat boys and sorority girls, both flirting away and gliding through school on daddy's money. Along with the 'Greeks' were the 'hippies,' a developing peace-loving group who demonstrated often outside the center. Outcasts with no particular affiliation, such as Edward, used the center to grab a bite to eat or catch a cat nap between classes. Today the duel purpose was fulfilled.

Partially satiated by the peanut butter and jelly, slopped heavily with both condiments then washed down with what the hippies had demonstrated to be contaminated water, Edward began to drift. Somewhere between a daydream and a nightmare he worried about the eight weeks remaining until finals. He had to make better use of his time or somehow scrape together more hours in every day.

His only option, aside from selling his body or drugs, or failing outright, lay nestled within the seven digits in his backpack. Squinting from the light, still partially dazed he looked around, pulled his pack closer, unzipped the worn out bag and reached in for the scrap. Memorizing the number he reinserted the paper, set his watch for ten minutes and grabbed some shut-eye before his next class. It was settled. Tonight, in the semi-privacy of his shared apartment, he would find out just how much a 'sperm bank' was willing to dish out for superior 'med student' sperm.

The evening came and his roommate was due home in less than twenty minutes. Without further procrastination he began dialing the number.

"Stanford Fertility Clinic. This is Marcia, can I help you?"
Her voice sounded young and spunky, not old and crotchety
as he had hoped, making his next words all the more difficult.
His professional response to her hello, which he had practiced
several times in front of his mirror, immediately escaped him.

"Um.... well, I was walking...and I noticed a bright orange
flyer...you know, the one on sp...sperm donation." Before
he had the chance to humiliate himself further with his
inarticulateness, the receptionist saved him with her matter-of-
fact, 'no big deal' approach. As if they were discussing the stock
market, she made him feel four notches more comfortable.

"Our usual procedure involves a brief consultation prior to
donation. I need to put you on hold while I get the appointment
book." With nerves rising, the thought of conversing about his
ejaculated sample or any related topic for that matter, began
to nauseate his entire being. He agreed to hold while he too
dropped the receiver to fetch his pocket calendar. Running back
to the phone then realizing he was without a pen, he stretched
the cord to reach a desk drawer. Tossing two empty pens in the
waste basket, he found a third one that actually contained ink.

"How does next Tuesday sound? Dr. Welter has openings at
either 1:00 or 2:30."

He flipped his calendar to view the following Tuesday, then
realized he had a lab that started at 2:00.

"The 1:00 will be fine. How much time should I allow?"
Edward jotted the entry into the corresponding time frame.

"A half hour is usual, unless you have a lot of questions. Can
I get your name?"

Realizing that he was committed from this point on he
spoke in a clear, concise fashion. "Edward Black."

"I assume you are a med student."

"Yes, second year."

The remainder of the conversation was a blur and was
over in a matter of minutes, completed just seconds before the
arrival of his nosy roommate.

❧

The week flew by. There was no time to dwell on Tuesday's appointment. He pulled into the clinic parking lot in his beat-up Plymouth, less than a mile from his apartment. Hoping that sweat or physical exertion would have no ill effect on the vitality of his sperm, he made a mental note to ride his bike to the "real" appointment. Climbing over the console and out the passenger door, the only one that opened, he headed toward the corresponding suite. In bold print next to suite 3B read: Sperm Donations/Inseminations. Wishing he could be invisible, he failed to remove his sunglasses as his only recourse upon entering the antiseptic-smelling environment. The woman behind the window appeared to be inundated with work. Her back was turned as she worked on papers that were scattered, covering her work space entirely.

"Excuse me, I believe I have a 1:00 appointment here today." Edward was proud that his almost whisper of a voice didn't crack and glad that only one other patient existed in the waiting room. He assumed he was speaking to Marcia, but really didn't care to ask.

Respecting his cue, Marcia lowered her voice as she spoke. "You must be Edward Black..." She paused, looking for a sign of affirmation. He nodded. "The doctor is running a little behind schedule. He will be with you shortly. In the mean time, would you mind filling out this questionnaire?" She handed him a clipboard with a form attached.

Eric felt the weight of the other patient's stare as he turned to take a seat. Briefly he met eyes with a young man about his age but quickly turned and began writing. Knowledge of family health history was sketchy at best. Nothing too riveting in the way of disease seemed to occur with his relatives. They all seemed to plug right along into their late seventies or early eighties before heart failure or cancer caught up with them. There was one exception he decided to omit from the questionnaire.

The door to the right of the reception window opened. A wimpy looking man entered the waiting area. Edward and the other patient looked up. His rounded shoulders were sadly apparent through his puckering white smock. His perfectly manicured hands gave away the fact that this man was probably the doctor. He was male, and that's all that mattered to Edward at the moment.

"Edward?" He waited for acknowledgment from either of the young men. Edward perked up, gathered the stapled forms and stood.

"Would you please follow me down the hall to my office?" The doctor presented his question more like an order. Edward seriously wondered if he was going to like the doc. He was then motioned to take a seat in his rather aesthetically decorated office. Skylights and a multitude of plants were clustered about, giving the office an 'airy' garden-like feel.

"I'm Dr. Welter. It's always a pleasure to meet a future physician." He scratched his balding head then grabbed a folder with blue stickers adhered to the upper left corner.

"Nice to meet you too." Edward managed to squeeze in a few cordial words before being overrun by the man in control. Dr. Welter reached for Edward's hand, but instead of shaking it he surprised Edward by taking the clipboard. He ran the forms through a three hole punch and stuck them in the folder. Edward was relieved to be spared the embarrassment of shaking hands when his palms were so sweaty.

"As I go over your profile will you help fill in the details?" Dr. Welter wasted no time getting to business.

"Sure." Edward wondered what more he could possibly want to know but was more than willing to answer any questions he may have in store.

Dr. Welter began by reviewing the health history portion of the questionnaire. His fingers slid quickly down the page, keeping in sync with previously checked boxes answered 'no' to diseases of the heart, blood and kidneys, not to mention cancers of all kinds. The doctor read the note regarding heart disease and cancer in Edward's older relatives and looked up.

"Well, Edward, seeing that your relatives live well into their seventies and eighties before their health failed them, it doesn't look like your health history will be an issue with you. As far as I can see, you seem to be the perfect candidate for sperm donation." He folded his arms, leaned back in his chair and looked Edward up and down.

"With your bone structure, build and brains, any woman should count herself lucky to receive your sperm."

Edward didn't know how to respond. He could feel himself blushing; his face turned bright red. Thankfully, Dr. Welter's eyes were focused on the questionnaire, allowing time for Edward's face to cool.

"Third year medical school, working three to four shifts a week. That must equate to at least twenty hours a week!"

"Sometimes up to thirty. "

"You must be exhausted?" He raised his eyes from under his spectacles and turned to face a cluster of bottled terrariums.

"Only on my good days!" Edward chuckled and Dr. Welter managed a smile.

"So I take it you're not here to contribute to the betterment of mankind?

Edward squirreled in his chair. "No, Doctor. Money is the sole reason for my presence today."

"I respect your honesty. You may donate twice, sometimes three or four times if our need increases. We'll be using fresh as well as frozen samples. Your first donation, along with a blood test, will be analyzed. We'll be looking mainly at sperm count and mobility as well as health problems associated with your blood. If found to be healthy, regular donations will be accepted." He paused then continued. "At this time, we are willing to pay twenty-five dollars for each donation." Eric's eyes lit up and his posture became erect.

"I was hoping this would be the answer to my problems." Edward reached over to shake the Doctor's hand and this time was met with a firm grip. "I take it I shouldn't quit my night job until after the 'sperm screening.' The word 'sperm' somehow rolled off his tongue with ease as he looked directly into the spectacles where the doctor's enlarged topaz-colored eyes stared back.

"You are correct, but I would predict a man of your age

and apparent health status will have not only an excellent sperm count, but vitality too. Why don't we take a sample now, and I could give you a call before, say...noon tomorrow?"

The words seemed to echo in slow motion. He was unprepared mentally for clinical ejaculation at this point in the game. A small, hardly noticeable pause overtook the plant-infested office before Edward responded with a nod.

He was led down a hallway and directed into a stark room. In the far corner was a stack of girly magazines which, at first, didn't help the lack of ambiance throughout the dungeon. In a nook to the right of the entrance sat a cup and a pamphlet detailing the steps involved in the creation of successful samples. As if men don't have experience with masturbation, Edward thought. A small sliding door was located behind the nook. Edward figured it led to the lab. He pictured millions, probably billions of other hopeful sperm waiting in their little cups.

"At least they don't make you walk around the office with your sample, yelling 'Nurse...Nurse, here's my sperm!" Edward muffled a laugh, realizing that someone might be in earshot.

Three times he wanted to throw in the towel, but something practical kept telling him it was his way out, his only choice if he was to pass this semester. He concentrated hard, picked up a magazine and got to work. A few minutes later he, an ounce lighter, was on his way.

The call came earlier then expected, while the shower was running. Noticing there were no towels in the bathroom, he swore, and headed directly for his roommate's room, or 'pig sty' as Edward referred to it, in search of used towels. Three donations a month and he wouldn't have to deal with this or any roommate, he thought.

He picked up on the fifth ring.

"Hello," Edward said, his voice still angered from the towel episode.

"May I speak to Edward Black?" He recognized Marcia's voice.

"This is he." Never before had he wished for healthy

sperm. On the contrary, he routinely hoped for deficient sperm equipped with the staying power of an eighty-five-year old man. This thought pattern, he believed, kept his "guys" from puncturing the big egg. Today was different. He crossed his fingers in hopes of healthy, strong and most importantly, lucrative sperm.

"This is Marcia from the Stanford Fertility Clinic. Did I catch you at a good time or should I call later?"

"I wasn't expecting you to call until noon, but this is fine." He held the phone between his shoulder and ear, wrapped the foul-smelling towel around his naked bottom half, then stretched the cord enough to shut off the shower.

"Your sperm has been analyzed and was found to be good quality. I have some forms that describe the procedures from here on out. Would you prefer to pick them up or shall I drop them in the mail this morning?" Edward's heart skipped a beat as he spoke, "Why don't I stop by after class today and save you the postage. How late are you open?"

"I'll be here until five, but I can leave it.... "

"My class is over at four. I'll see you shortly after. "

"O.K. See you then."

FOURTEEN

Three Months *Later*

Beatrice Clooney had worked at the clinic for a mere six months but kept up with the status of all Dr. Welter's patients. The doctors loved her and Marcia could see how quickly people had grown to respect her work. Beatrice was personable with the staff and the patients and absolutely fell in love with all the babies after delivery. Her perky personality filled with endless enthusiasm and good humor was really beginning to wear on Marcia. In fact, it was enough to make Marcia green with envy!

"I really hope the Edwards are successful this time." Beatrice realized conversation with Marcia was futile. She expressed her feelings anyway, despite the fact that she happened to be standing next to her least favorite person at the clinic as the Edwards passed.

"Can't say we didn't do our best to make it happen." Marcia's reply was short and cool.

Beatrice let the comment roll right off, nodded and decided to let it go when Marcia chimed in again.

"Were you aware that this was the Edwards' last chance this round at a biological child?" Marcia continued to flaunt her expertise on the personal aspects and seemingly vast knowledge of office procedures. Beatrice Clooney, as a fairly new employee, would have had no exposure to nor opportunity to have witnessed some of the behind the scenes procedures that Marcia was referring to. Miss Clooney's expression confirmed her curiosity and obvious ignorance on the subject, which was exactly Marcia's intention.

"Last chance,...what do you mean by that?" Beatrice, her patience wearing, managed to hold strong her failing sincerity.

"I should just hand you the chart so you can nose around on your own, but since I have a minute, I may as well explain to you how things work around here." Marcia was eating up the moment as she flipped her unruly hair, reapplied the red lipstick that matched her fingernail polish, then grabbed the Edwards chart and continued. "You may think your job as a nurse is, aside from the doctor, the most important. Sure, you talk to the patient, make them feel comfortable and take their blood pressure every once in a while." If it was possible to feel one's own blood pressure rise, Beatrice could swear hers was beginning to soar. Still she only nodded, aware that it was worthless to get even with a person made of such substandard material. She continued to listen to the long winded airhead, in hopes that she would eventually get to the point.

"The detailed and most intricate work goes on before the insemination is even performed. Dr. Welter and I, well...actually our families, go way back. I can't tell you how many times he's declared how absolutely indispensable I am as his number one employee. I've been here since he started this practice, and he has taught me almost everything about the back office, the lab, as well as the front office." Marcia left herself wide open and Beatrice couldn't waste the opportunity to give her just one small jab.

"Are you eventually going to discuss the Edwards and some of these procedures of extreme importance?" Marcia's face went red and a vein in her forehead began to pulsate. As she spoke her voice began to quiver with anger.

"If you would show me some of the patience you seem to have on hand for the doctors and patients, I will get to them." Marcia looked a little frazzled as she spoke, giving Beatrice time to dwell on the moment.

"Are you O.K., Marcia?" Beatrice motioned at something near or on Marcia's face. "There is sweat all over your nose, and you look a bit rosy. Maybe I should take your blood pressure?"

"I'm fine, and as I was saying, my job entails more than you medical people give me credit for. After the thorough screening that I must administer prior to the medical examination, I organize each and every chart according to procedure." Beatrice was sickened at the way Marcia loved to hear herself speak.

"The chart is only the tip of the iceberg. The lab is my next undertaking. The six vials must be meticulously labeled and set out for you, I assume. Each vial will eventually contain the sperm of the donor and represents one round at artificial insemination. Most clinics only give the poor couple one or two chances,...not us." She paused once again, after rambling aimlessly about every office procedure she could pull from her small mind.

"Are you able to grasp most of this information and relate it to the Edwards, or do I need to spell it out?" Before Beatrice could respond, Marcia and her self-centered personality overrode any comment Beatrice may have used for a reply. "To make a long story short, Brick Edwards was on his last vial." She opened the chart, flipped through it then held it out towards Beatrice.

"See, you can see the entries regarding the insemination attempts. We even go to the trouble of numbering each attempt with this color coded numbering system. Dr. Welter was amazed when I came up with that idea! You see, I'm basically in charge of the samples from the time they are filled, to the time they are 'dispensed', so to speak." She ran her hand through her hair then pointed her arrogant finger to the last entry dated today. A purple sticker labeled with a six was adhered neatly beside the progress notes regarding the insemination.

"See, I just finished sticking this in his chart...and you probably thought all I did up here is answer the phone and file my nails."

"Very impressive." Beatrice remarked in a sarcastic tone. Beatrice turned and walked back towards the lab. "Thank you so much for your valuable time, Marcia." This comment was said underneath her breath and most likely out of ear shot, but felt good just the same. She pushed at the white, swinging double doors of the lab, then made a mental note to unravel all there was to know about the lab and the employees authorized to work inside.

She turned around, left the lab as quickly as she entered, walked to the exam rooms and checked to see if Dr. Welter was ready for the swarm of patients expected this afternoon. For the first time, she began to question the exorbitantly high success rate at the clinic. The studies she read in school had a much lower success rate, but, with Marcia dabbling with the lab she suspected the possibility of foul play. Why was Marcia, possessing at best a high school diploma, given so much responsibility? Beatrice knew Marcia's qualifications were best suited for the front office. Why was she allowed to work in the lab, and given free rein in organizational procedures dealing with such delicate matters? One glance at the front office and one would immediately conclude that organization was far from Marcia's strong suit.

Having worked seven years in this office and obtaining the title of office manager was still not enough to satiate her need for power and recognition. No, Marcia needed more to offset the attention her new 'enemy' was receiving. Marcia and Dr. Welter seemed close, which presented another problem. Beatrice realized she needed to be discreet in her snooping.

She dreaded the nights she closed the clinic, but after her midday chat with Marcia, Beatrice had developed a rejuvenation, so to speak, for her late shifts. It was past eight-thirty and the last of many patients were leaving. She knew it would be only a matter of minutes before Dr. Welter would follow. She busied herself with paper work and placed an extra stack of files on her desk strictly for effect.

"Miss Clooney, shall I walk you to your car?" She looked up from the words she heard every time she worked late, and responded this time with a rehearsed reply.

"By the looks of it I'll be here until morning!" She was hoping she sounded natural and that she hadn't overdone it with the mountain of files precariously sitting to her right.

Motioning to the files, Dr. Welter said, "You work too hard, Beatrice. Can't you get to those in the morning?" He looked sincere, but she was determined to pull off her stunt.

"Have you checked out the schedule for tomorrow, or for the rest of the week for that matter?" She was willing to give in, if he pushed leaving again.

Instead he picked up his briefcase that he had placed beside her desk and replied, "I made it a point when I started the clinic. I look at the schedule the morning of, and not before. It makes for a more restful night, I've found." He reached for his keys in coin-filled pockets, by the sound of it, as he continued in his matter-of-fact, unsuspecting tone. "Be careful, Beatrice...see you tomorrow."

As soon as she heard the purr of his Mercedes round the corner, she hurried into the lab. She knew the cleaning crew would arrive soon, so she went to work on her ambiguous hunch.

The cryopreservation door was equipped with a lock, rarely engaged, from her observation on the rare occasion she spent in the lab. Vials upon vials, filled with sperm, sat in neat rows in the freezer. Taking a closer look, Beatrice noted sets of six with duplicate labels adhered to the side of each vial.

Goosebumps covered her exposed arms and the better part of her legs that were scantily covered by a thin layer of white nursing stockings. Without clearly knowing why or what she was looking for, Beatrice began scanning the neatly lined vials for some sort of alphabetizing, or system of arrangement. The chilling temperature was beginning to make her hands numb and her nose run. She spotted Eddison, Eddy, then six blank slots followed by Fergusen and Fernando. She suspected the Edwards slots would be empty and had proved absolutely nothing to her undetermined hypothesis. Closing the freezer, Beatrice moved onto the counter area to her left that housed numerous petri dishes, color coded to signify the developmental stage of the eggs and sperm. The cupboards above were filled with medical supplies and office paraphernalia, some of which were foreign to Beatrice, all of which were tossed haphazardly on any convenient shelf and in no particular order. Funny, Beatrice thought; aside from the labeling and color coding, with Marcia's command both the front office and lab were in a deep disarray. She couldn't help but wonder how a clinic so disorganized could be so incredibly successful.

In the midst of her exploration she heard the jingle of keys from the front office entrance, which abruptly broke her train of thought. Relieved to hear Al, alone tonight, cheerfully whistling, as he usually does, Beatrice whisked her hand through her disheveled hair and made an attempt to regain her usual composure.

Without satisfying her curiosity, she closed the cupboard, walked toward the lab door and refastened the barrette that was now dangling loosely in her silky hair. She tilted her head in such a way that a sparkle, coming from the trash dispenser, caught her eye and instantly filled her with intrigue. It looked like a vial. She paused, then realized she had run out of time and continued toward the door only to meet Al head on, dust mop and all.

"Give me a minute...I never forget a pretty face." Al stopped only to take a better look at Beatrice, who was blushing a bit from his comment, before he continued to reacquaint himself with her. "It's the name I admit to having trouble with, and yours is on the tip of my tongue."

Beatrice managed a smile, hoping her guilt wasn't evident around the edges. "It's Beatrice, Al. Nice to see you again." Turning back towards the petri dishes she continued, "Uh. . I'll be done in here in just a minute." Al seemed to get the hint right away. He reached down and picked up his plastic bucket full of cleaning supplies.

"Not a problem Bea, I'll simply start up front."

"Thank you Al. "

"Busy day, I take it." Al backed his way out of the lab and made his way toward the disarray of the front office.

"Yeah, worse than usual. "

As soon as the coast was clear Beatrice went straight for the trash dispenser. She crouched, pulled the liner and all from the dispenser, set it down, opened the cupboard above it, found the refill bags, relined the trash container and was ready to make a break for the bathroom when she realized Al might find it strange to discover the trash emptied. A nervous giggle unexpectedly erupted from her lips when she realized how totally paranoid she was acting. Nevertheless, she'd seen one too many detective movies and was bound and determined to cover her tracks. She opened up the trash and transferred some unworthy evidence such as used paper towels, Dixie cups and other paper products of no value to her hunch. Marcia spoke of vials. Vials interested Beatrice. Setting the trash beside the door of the lab, Beatrice walked toward her desk to check on Al's progress. He was busy Windexing the window that separated the front office and the waiting room. She opened her office drawer, seized her purse then briskly walked back to the lab, picked up the valuable trash, stuffed it into her purse and darted into the single stall bathroom. She turned on the light and locked the door simultaneously.

As she rummaged through the trash she confirmed the sparkling object to be one of seven vials. The glass from the vials must have been the culprit. She carefully lifted the vials and gently lined them upon the floor, for what reason she wasn't sure. She reached inside her purse in search of paper, pulled a checkbook deposit slip from behind her checks, scrambled for a pen and began jotting down the names and label color for each vial.

"Beatrice, are you done in the lab?" Al broke his happy whistling session to shout these words.

Startled, but far from "uncool," Beatrice replied, "Yes, Al, thanks for asking. I'll be leaving shortly." The whistling started up and Beatrice resumed her list.

Sitting on the yet to be disinfected bathroom floor, straddling a mound of trash, Beatrice worked fast. Her adrenaline temporarily soared when she recovered a vial labeled Edward Black, but no vial labeled Brick Edwards had turned up as she began replacing the trash inside the liner. The first heap she tossed back included a soda can. Upon impact the can

clinked with a hard object. Half disgusted with herself, Beatrice
reentered the scum infested liner and poked around to find one
last vial. This one, for some reason, was wrapped loosely in a
paper towel. Right away she noticed the unusual weight of the
vial. As she unwrapped the specimen, she gasped and cupped
her hand over her face to muffle the sound. The vial was filled
with semen. The label read 'Brick Edwards.'

    As she headed on Highway 101, leaving Stanford, she was
still shaken by her findings. Why would a full vial be tossed?
Why wasn't Brick Edwards last sample used? Confusion began
to fog her usually clear thought pattern. What to do with her
new-found information, or who she could trust with it were
part of plan B, something Beatrice hadn't put much thought
into yet. An accusation of tampering with lab specimens could
mean the end of Dr. Welter's career as well as Marcia's and the
other doctors affiliated with the practice. The clinic would
surely close and she would also be jobless, and hated for that
matter. Beatrice loved her job, the money being far better than
a 'non-specialty' staff nurse in a hospital, not to mention the
decent shifts she was pulling now. Yes, comparing herself to
nursing friends, she had the red carpet treatment. After all, Dr.
Welter was making it possible for childless couples to become
families. Why though, was Brick Edwards' vial, thought to be
used last month, tossed in today's trash?

    The auto pilot button was abruptly turned off as she pulled
into her carport. Without really realizing it, Beatrice had talked
herself out of a confrontation and had given herself permission
to hold her tongue in this matter.

    The pictures of the infants filled the walls completely, and
as Silvia glanced up, she noticed that in the last three weeks the
ceiling had become fair game for display. Pamphlets answering
every possible question on artificial insemination were stacked
on tables. The wealth of information was surrounded by plants,
in bottle terrariums. Dr. Welter explained the significance of

the plants in one of their initial meetings. His words rang in her head every time she entered the familiar office.

"New life and growth is a miracle. Just give me the seeds of life to germinate. I will plant them in their natural habitat. If the seed is nurtured the miracle of life will endure."

The renowned Dr. Welter worked on the cutting edge. He was a master at the creation of life, as was evident in both the glass jars and the wombs of many women. This office always made her feel optimistic about their chances of conception.

Hands folded and head down, Brick sat motionless in the chair next to his second wife, Silvia. He had great hopes of the procedure taking, but with last month constituting their sixth attempt, discouraging thoughts surfaced.

Waiting for Dr. Welter to be the bearer of bad news, once again made him feel both depressed and anxious. He tried to grasp the situation by deep breathing and focusing on only positive outcomes.

The silence and privacy in the office only amplified the tension. Silvia couldn't take another minute of it. She broke the silence by voicing her thoughts.

"I really do feel different this time, Brick." She nudged him with her right hand to stir him from his partial trance.

Brick turned, locked eyes with her and reached for her hand. "So do I," he said, trying to rid the desperation from his voice and instead sound supportive.

"No, really I feel a bit nauseated, and more tired than usual." She was speaking with true conviction. "And just look at this!" At this point she pulled her sweater off her shoulders and exposed her newly developed voluptuousness. "I think they have increased at least a cup size."

Brick's eyes bulged with astonishment as they dropped from her eyes to her chest. "When did this all happen?" He reached out to touch her swelling breasts that were covered only by a thin cotton blouse. "I cant' believe I didn't notice."

She intercepted and warned, "Be gentle. They are so incredibly sore and have been for at least a week. I wanted to tell you before, but was afraid I'd get your hopes up."

Brick's eyes immediately began to fill with tears of joy. He steered his reach from her breast to the back of her shoulder and leaned in for a squeeze when the door opened slightly. Modestly, they resumed upright positions in their chairs.

The sound of the chart being taken from its slot on the back of the door preceded the brief rumbling between Dr. Welter and a nurse. He entered his office, held out a hand for Brick to shake and Silvia to gain reassurance from. His hands were always a little clammy and were connected to rather wimpy looking appendages that intersected with rounded shoulders and a sunken chest. All in all his self esteem, at least in his work environment, was not effected by his physical inadequacies.

He sat with chart in hand, looked up at the anxious couple, smiled and began speaking. "I'm happy to inform you both that the artificial insemination procedure was successful." He paused, as if to take pleasure in the precious moment that couldn't have taken place without him. He continued, "The pregnancy test was positive and the exam conducted today confirms to us that you are three weeks into you first trimester.

Brick and Silvia were stunned. Hearing the doctor say the words was music to their ears. Brick stood to shake Dr. Welter's hand then immediately reached for his pregnant wife. He turned only to see tears of joy streaming down her beautiful face. Her clear complexion was slightly blotchy with emotion as her eyes sparkled all the more with abundant tears. Her light brown hair was sleek, almost radiant, with the ends curled up in the latest style.

"This is unbelievable," she exclaimed, as she too turned and reached up for Brick's hand. "Will everything be normal from here on out?" She blotted her tears, trying not to smear her mascara.

"Of course there are no guarantees with any pregnancy, and I will recommend the normal precautions that should be taken by any woman in her first trimester. Other than that, I feel we should have a very predictable pregnancy with the normal complaints that I'm sure you'll be experiencing very soon if you haven't already."

Welter rolled his chair to his desk, leafed through a file and pulled from it two well-worn articles. "Here, before you leave, make sure you get a photocopy." He reached across his desk and placed the current literature in front of the ecstatic couple. "If you are interested in any worthwhile books on pregnancy, take a look at the bibliography for some excellent resources. If you have any questions or concerns, please don't hesitate to call." He stood, as if to prompt Brick and Silvia to the conclusion of the appointment. Brick and Silvia followed his lead out of the serene office back out to the busy reception area. Dr. Welter stopped when he reached the counter which faced the patients directly through the window. This particular area seemed to emulate the hub of "Grand Central Station." He scribbled something on a prescription pad, handed it to Silvia and said, "Here is a prescription for prenatal vitamins. Start taking one a day."

Silvia nodded then inquired, "Will I be notified of my next appointment, or should I go ahead and schedule it now?"

"Marcia can make you a photocopy and schedule an appointment in six weeks. He was walking backwards and, as usual, in a hurry.

His rushing through their appointments had become almost expected to Brick and Silvia. At first, before conception, Dr. Welter's rather brief manner combined with the general disarray in the clinic, was frustrating. Today, on the other hand, nothing could bother the happy couple, even if half of Silvia's inheritance was already in Dr. Welter's pocket. After all, without his expertise, a growing fetus would undoubtedly not be present in Silvia's nurturing womb. They left The Stanford Fertility Clinic ecstatic.

FIFTEEN

Eight Months *Later*

The waiting room was suffocating, with the heat penetrating like there was no tomorrow. Brick had even found himself dozing twice, felt guilty, then walked down the dismal hallway for more of the stale coffee from the vending machine. The four hours felt like ten. Kenny and Mitchell seemed to come much faster, but with his new knowledge on the subject of labor and delivery, he was very aware of the individual differences in every delivery, especially from one woman to the next.

A much younger man, in his late teens or early twenties, entered the waiting 'chamber' roughly an hour after Brick's arrival. His bowed legs paced continuously in his Wranglers and clattering cowboy boots, making it all the more difficult to relax. Not a word had been spoken between them yet. Brick finally broke the silence.

"So...are you hoping for a boy or a girl?"

The young lad did not respond initially, leading Brick to believe that conversation would be nonexistent with this obvious country-western fan. Brick had all but given up when the young man turned and began speaking in a Southern drawl. His words were slow and deliberate and a pleasure to Brick's ears.

"Well...since we have a little girl at home waiting for us, I'm more inclined towards a boy, to carry on the family name and all."

As he spoke, his youth, or rather unworldliness, surfaced

with a simple, less than confident southern drawl. His pacing went unaltered as he continued his rather warm, 'open book' style with his new acquaintance. "I'm so nervous I could scream. You'd think I'd be better this time around, but no...my wife has to go through so much pain...I can't stand it...Here I am rambling about myself, and here you are going through the same thing. You'll have to excuse my manners, sir. Is this your first?"

Brick, feeling better with the light conversation, answered, "I have two sons from a previous marriage. This is my second wife's first." A perplexed look came over the Southern boy. The expression changed to a smile as they both chuckled at Brick's previous wording. Brick continued speaking, moving his eyes from the young lad to a void on the wall as he concentrated on the comment at hand.

"I agree with you, it does seem to get harder. I think the whole ordeal would be a lot easier if they would let us out of this 'dungeon' and actually allow us to participate in the delivery."

True panic struck the Southern boy's face. "Oh no, I couldn't listen to all the moaning...and the blood...have you heard how much blood comes out? No, thank you! I'd much rather do my suffering in here!"

Brick, trying to avoid hitting another raw nerve, steered the conversation back to the post-delivery portion of babyhood. "Do you have any names picked out?"

The boy's look of panic was replaced by an ear-to-ear grin.

"If it's a girl my wife likes Lisa and I like James, Jr., after his father, if it's a boy." Young James looked very proud and self involved at the finish of his sentence. He drifted momentarily to some rather personal thoughts while Brick pretended not to notice the break in the conversation. After the brief intermission and for the first time in over an hour, a pause in his pacing, James spoke again. "Do you have a name for your little tyke?"

Brick was taken by surprise, thinking the conversation had again died. He woke from his daydream and replied in a monotone. "Eric if it's a boy, Erica if it's a girl."

"Well, let me shake your hand...uh," he realized he didn't even know this man's name.

"I'm Brick, nice to meet you, James." Brick reached, shook and was met with an abundantly masculine grip.

"My little one is Erica, too; a fine name if I do say so myself!" He chuckled again, exposing a missing molar space on his upper right side. "It's really nice to make your acquaintance, Brick."

The handshake disengaged as the double doors to the waiting room were pushed open to expose a woman, clad entirely in white. Matching booties covered her shoes and she wore what appeared to be a white shower cap on her head.

"Mr. Edwards?" she said as she glanced, first in Brick's direction and then towards James.

Brick's face lit up. "Yes, is everything all right?" He stood and walked to greet her. She smiled and he immediately was overcome with a combination of relief and excitement.

"Congratulations. You are the father of a healthy baby boy. Dr. Welter is just finishing the suturing. You're welcome to come and take a look in just a few minutes. "

The nurse in white turned to James. "The last I checked, your wife's labor was moving right along." She gave him reassuring eye contact and a comforting smile. "It shouldn't be much longer." She turned, closed the door and left the two men to their emotions.

In addition to the firm grip, Brick's back received a series of light pats, progressively gaining velocity and finally concluded with an inescapable embrace that Brick surrendered to. "Congratulations my friend. You must feel as happy as a range fed Holstein!" Brick stepped back to avoid a second embrace.

"You hit the nail right on the head," Brick replied, almost chuckling at his choice of words.

"Well 'git' on in there now. Go kiss that son of yours." Brick noticed the tears welling up in James' eyes as Brick turned to greet his infant. Pretending not to notice as he held back his own, he took one last look at him and straight from his heart said, "It was great to meet you, James."

"Likewise, likewise."

SIXTEEN

Thirty Years *Later*

The sun was setting as Eric watched Amanda sleep on their checkered picnic blanket that had been placed strategically, downwind from the Cheese Factory. The grassy knoll that overlooked the duck pond was partially hidden from the backroads and was nestled between two ancient oaks. The continuous conversation started shortly after their good-byes to Tiny and Jim and a handful of calls to cancel the day's appointments, and continued through until a short while ago.

Eric was tempted to wake her, but with her eyelids moving and busy, waking her would mean taking her away from what appeared to be a wonderful dream. Instead, Eric reached for Amanda's purse and pulled out his cellular phone. Grabbing a partially gnawed-on bagel that lay beside her purse, he headed toward a picnic table that sat adjacent to the pond. Pinching off, then tossing tidbits of bagel flesh in the water, he watched the rings form around the morsels. The circumference grew with time until the flurry of ducks and geese broke through the forming rings, spoiling the perfect circles with their own wake. The ganders flocked around him, demanding morsels of their own. Walking back to the blanket with new friends in tow, Eric picked up the remaining bagels, stood on the far corner of the blanket and within a blink of an eye, the bag was empty. Amazingly enough the noisy gluttons didn't arouse the slightest stir, as Amanda continued in her deep slumber. Flipping back the cellular, he dialed his way out of a dinner consisting of a multitude of stinky cheeses. Relieved, the directory connected him to Round Table Pizza in Novato. With promise of a sizable tip, he ordered a medium vegetarian, light on the cheese.

The begging flock took over the blanket. When they realized their food source was gone, they moved on to better prospects. Fifteen minutes passed. Eric sat Indian-style on the grass beside the blanket. Carefully rethinking the day's events and attempting to recapture and store every detail, he sat on the limited poop-free area, available beside the blanket. It was the silence, or the lack of quacking, that pulled her back to the conscious world. Her eyes opening to Eric's stare startled Amanda. Dazed and slightly confused, she sat up, looked around and began speaking, voice cracking and raspy like the morning.

"What time is it?" She rubbed her eyes then forced them to open a little wider.

"You've been sleeping for about forty-five minutes. Just nodded off in the middle of my story. I think you started snoring on my tenth birthday. So I assume you left off when I was nine or so!" His sarcasm left them both smiling as Amanda lay back down to catch the last bit of the sun disappearing over the horizon. She stretched her arms over her head, yawned, then screamed.

"Oh, my God...what's all over my arms?" She displayed to Eric numerous splotches of greenish brown duck poop on her arms and hands.

"The bagel-eating monsters just left your side. I thought for sure you would wake up. Instead I see they left you gifts!"

"You let them poop all over my blanket...you ass!" Looking around she realized the blanket and surrounding areas were pretty well splattered with slimy fowl droppings.

The pizza delivery couldn't have come at a better time. Eric ran for the parking lot, tipped the kid a twenty, grabbed some extra napkins and started back toward Amanda. As he jolted, close enough to be heard, he began begging for forgiveness. He reached the now overturned blanket in record time, then proceeded to kneel and continue his prideless plea. "My darling and devoted wife...in return for my thoughtless act of wasting the last of your hearty bagels and letting the ducks have their way with your precious blanket, I have brought, in exchange, a doughy conglomerate covered with cheeses and vegetables. Please take this and accept my apology. Please...anything but the guillotine and I will be your slave until eternity!"

Laughing, she walked toward him then quickly turned away after snitching the small stack of napkins sitting on top of the pizza box.

"I'll contemplate that while I remove the dung from my extremities...slave!" She walked toward the pond to moisten the napkins in the lake as Eric enjoyed his view from behind.

The cool water felt refreshing as she wiped her arms and hands. She was tempted to slosh her face then decided against it as the ducks and geese appeared out of nowhere, quacking and undoubtedly pooping. Still in a very relaxed state she made her way back to the blanket that had been tossed aside. Eric, who began to inhale his second piece, had re-situated on a nearby picnic table.

"Aren't slaves supposed to wait until their masters have eaten, before indulging?" She joined him and took in the purple and pink swirls of the dusk sky.

"Oh, I guess I forgot to tell you. I was referring to strictly... a sex slave." Taking time out from the constant shoving in of food, he turned to catch her reaction.

Helping herself to a piece she managed to keep a straight face. She turned and spoke. "I can only imagine how you will suffer when I chain you to the bed. So selfless to think of yourself as a slave!"

"Sex every night...I can visualize the horror and can only imagine the demands put upon my maleness." He paused as he caught the array of visual possibilities, turning his stare to a smirk.

"Are you insinuating that our bedtime ritual leaves you less than satisfied? Is that what this is all about?" More alert now, her tone turned serious as she propped herself up with her elbows.

"That's just it...a ritual. Wham, bam, thank you...Eric. I need more cuddling and caressing. My heart rate hardly has a chance to return to normal and you've already turned over and resumed where your last dream took off."

"I guess I have been a little sluggish lately. It's just that I'm so tired. Last Thursday for instance. It's as if I have narcolepsy. Did I tell you I had to pull over and rest on my way to Sacramento last week?"

"No. "Concern entered his expression.

"I knew if I didn't close my eyes willingly, they would have done so without my permission. I napped on Highway 80 for almost a half hour. "

"Maybe you're running too hard. I know you've been working hard on increasing your pace."

"Yeah, I thought about that too. I haven't changed my running schedule for over a year, except for the extra track workout, which I doubt could account for the exhaustion. Maybe this is the way people feel in their mid-thirties?" Sarcasm entered her tone.

"Maybe you should get it checked out." Scratching his head, Eric squinted as he dabbled with his memory. "Didn't you tell me that Sally went through a tired spell last year? Didn't she finally go to the doctor to find out she was anemic? I know first hand how anemia can pull you down."

"Yeah, you're right, I'm long over due for a physical." With a sigh a relief she reached toward the pizza and selected three pieces that were adhered together. Placing two napkins under the slab she looked toward Eric. "I know...I know, I'm such a dainty eater! This way, I can admit to having only one piece before I fill up!"

"As long as it gives you the energy for commanding your personal slave.... and no, I'm not complaining. Maybe a little concerned with your lack of energy and enthusiasm lately, but not complaining."

"I'll call the doctor first thing in the morning to schedule an appointment. In the meantime I think I'll get in touch with Sally to see exactly what was ailing her last year."

SEVENTEEN

One Month *Later*

The doctor waved Amanda into his office prior to the actual exam. The long hallway needed updating, not to mention better ventilation. The colors of the tarnished walls were virtually indistinguishable and perfectly coordinated with the worn linoleum. The few pictures that hung on the walls most likely had their heyday in the early seventies. Stacks of files were precariously placed beside the reception area next to the office that she was to spend the initial portion of her physical exam. The place was far from fancy, but the doctor had a wonderful reputation.

She entered the small overcrowded office to find an empty chair facing his desk that she assumed was designated for patients. She took a minute to look around the office.

Yellowed pictures, drawn by young children, were taped haphazardly about. Assuming the artistic display was his children's work, she browsed and found a progression of family photographs in neat little frames on a table beside his desk. Two children, a boy and girl, were shown from infanthood up to what appeared to be their high school graduation. His wife, a natural beauty, aged ever so gracefully as the years brought her babies into adulthood.

The doctor entered and took a seat. Looking back towards the doctor as he began to speak, Amanda realized that he, too, had hardly aged in the past two decades. A little graying on the sideburns and the presence of a more chiseled face with laugh lines deepened, distinguished his rugged, good looks all the more.

"We need to discuss one issue before I forge ahead with a barrage of questions." He hesitated, noticed Amanda's anxiety rise along with her eyebrows and before further ado put the issue on the table. "Can you tell me the date of your last period?" With pen in hand and eyes securely adhered to hers, he waited for a reply.

A puzzled look came over Amanda. "Are the results showing that I'm pregnant? There must be a mistake...hold on." She reached in and dug through her purse to find her Day Runner. She flipped back a couple of weeks in search of the symbol she had used since she became sexually active, signifying the first day of her period. She found a little 'P' in red ink, scribbled in its usual spot on the lower right corner on Tuesday, September fourth. Relieved that she had, in fact, had her period two weeks prior, she looked up and answered.

"September fourth." She even went as far as to face her calendar in his direction to show where she had jotted the 'P.'

Acknowledging weakly with an ever so slight nod of his head, he began firing the next series of questions her way. All of the questions related to the early September period and basically gave him a blow by blow, detailed analysis of everything she could remember about the uneventful few days.

"Well, it was on the light side." Amanda retorted. She continued as doubt began to enter the picture. "My periods in the last year or two have been a little irregular...About the same time the true meaning of PMS has entered the picture, giving me no reason to worry with my light period, or the exhaustion."

The doctor, a little too clinical for her liking, looked up from his note taking to add some more matter-of-fact comments to the conversation. "Of course, we can't be absolutely sure, not without further tests, but a fair percentage of women spot in the first trimester and some throughout their pregnancies. With your cooperation I'd like my nurse practitioner to administer those tests and I'll try to contact an obstetrician from upstairs to administer a sonogram."

Like clockwork, lacking much emotional acknowledgment, the conversation was moved to the next topic at hand—the rest of her physical being. From system to system they marched, looking back on family history and childhood diseases. Nothing too noteworthy existed in her health history with exception of a great aunt on her father's side. The doctor hardly flinched and said the genes were too far removed to warrant any worry of passing such traits to offspring of her own. Amanda apparently asked one too many questions on the topic of albinism. The tangent she regarded as important only seemed to annoy him as he attempted to get back on track with questions regarding the present. Still she couldn't erase the visual of her Great Aunt Glenda, her pink eyes, transparent skin and hair, white as snow.

Now with the possibility of being pregnant, for the first time the worry of transmitting such a flawed helix made her stomach turn. A pit stop at the Civic Center Library was a must on today's agenda.

An hour later all tests, including the sonogram, proved positive for pregnancy. It was happening too fast and the excitement was almost more than Amanda could bear. Leaving the doctor's office shocked and in a fog, she drove on automatic pilot directly to Eric's office to find his desk vacant. Aware of the life growing inside her she felt dizzy and weak, not to mention hungry enough to gnaw on a piece of cardboard. She collapsed into his comfortable swivel chair and looked at the clock. Only eleven forty. Too ravenous to make it even to the Quick Mart across the street, she forced herself from the chair and walked across the office to the small kitchen area that housed a tiny refrigerator, microwave, coffee and espresso machines, miniature butcher block and table for two. Black spots distorted her vision, but still she was able to catch a glimpse of some sumptuous baked goods toward the rear of the fridge. It was then, with her arm inside the fridge reaching for what appeared to be homemade bread, that she met up with

Eric's secretary. Feeling as if she was caught red-handed with her hand in the cookie jar, she quickly threw the bread back on the shelf and closed the refrigerator while her face turned two shades of red.

"Hi Amanda,. . if it's bread you want, all you have to do is ask!" Smiling, Tina was completely sarcastic and was obviously trying to give her boss's wife a hard time. Amanda sat as the color of embarrassment faded, along with the black spots in her vision.

"Hasn't Eric warned you about my weakness for baked goods? I can't be trusted and can't be responsible for my behavior...especially now."

Tina, slicing the bread and slathering a delicious cream cheese concoction on two of the slices, was always up for a chat and absolutely thrived on gossip or 'juicy scoop,' as she referred to it.

"My ears are itching. I detect an interesting topic opening up? What's the saying...never a free lunch?" The twinkle in her eye was just the beginning of her overt curiosity in all matters of the soul.

Sinking her teeth and inhaling a whopping bite Amanda pondered the idea of telling all, then stopped herself. "You'll find out soon enough. It's really premature to mention at this point anyway." Pausing only to gulp the diet soda, Amanda continued to wolf down the bread.

"Diet sodas aren't recommended for pregnant women." With exception to the slight smirk, Tina held a straight face with eyes that exhibited x-ray vision.

Looking first at the soda then up to Tina, with a look that told all, Amanda stood, as did Tina, for an embrace of true congratulatory magnitude. It was then that Eric entered the picture.

"This must be some pretty "juicy" gossip. Whaddah miss?" Without really checking for subtleties, he reached for a soda, popped the top, gulped down three quarters of it, paused and realized he was being stared at by his two favorite women.

"I'll leave you two alone," Tina said, as she gave Amanda's hand one last squeeze before her departure.

By the looks of things Eric had concluded the news to be neither good or bad. With his thirst seemingly insatiable, he again lifted the soda to his lips and poured the remainder down, simultaneously opening the refrigerator for a second soda. Wiping the splash of soda from his chin he then leaned toward Amanda and kissed her on the mouth.

"So, what brings you to my office in the middle of the day?...not to mention unannounced, throwing my schedule into a tizzy?" He coaxed her from the chair and pressed his body close as he took in her scent.

Her arms wrapped around his lean torso with ease as she whispered, "I just got back from my doctor's appointment."

Guilty for forgetting her morning call and checkup, Eric took a step back as he placed both hands on Amanda's shoulders. "Everything went O.K.?"

Smiling, Amanda replied, "Let's just say the prognosis is shocking—but I'm fine."

"Something unexpected came up?"

While Amanda deliberately paused, Eric stood perplexed while he searched her face and his mind for what she was getting at.

"We are going to have a baby."

Shocked, he remained motionless. Before he realized what he was doing he had Amanda scooped up like an infant as he twirled her in excitement. A vase in their path was struck by Amanda's foot and was catapulted into the refrigerator where it shattered into many pieces on impact. Tina, alarmed at the noise, came running, peeked around the corner and witnessed Eric wiping tears of joy from Amanda's face. He too was crying and laughing and both were in their own world, completely oblivious to the eyes peering at this intimate moment. Realizing the broken vase must have been an accident, she left them, touched by the romance and passion of the scene.

The next three months came as a complete struggle for Amanda, with severe nauseousness that felt like the worst case of flu she had ever encountered. Bread and water were the only foods that didn't repulse her and calmed the rumbling in her stomach. Fresh brewed coffee, once a smell she cherished, caused the gag reflex on the first inhalation. Sleeping much, canceling and rescheduling appointments and basically existing in a fog were some things she wouldn't miss as she begin to pull away from the first trimester.

Entering her fourth month Amanda felt rejuvenated, less green and ready to eat anything thrown her way. Twisted french fries became a favorite for a few weeks until the pleasure of soft-serve ice cream, topped with chocolate chips and butterscotch syrup, prevailed. The smell of coffee, still not a pleasure, appealed to her from the perspective of caffeine, and the knowledge of its powerful benefits. Her doctor assured her that coffee consumed in moderation had been shown in no study to harm the baby. She laughed out loud when she recalled the definition of moderation that he had quoted from a recent study.

"Make sure you keep your consumption under six cups a day and you should be fine." Not even in the midst of finals did she ever consume a 'moderate' six cups in a twenty-four hour period.

All in all, things were looking up and growing outward in leaps and bounds according to the scale. Today's appointment reinforced that eating lots equated directly with weight gain. Some would rationalize the eight-pound increase to be the baby and related gestational factors. Amanda, who believed the formation of cellulite an impossibility on someone such as herself, had a rude awakening.

"I see you're feeling better, Amanda?" The doctor said with a smile. "Are you drinking lots of water?"

"I could probably do better." She felt a little disgusted, not to mention embarrassed, with her lack of control and motivation these days.

"Aim for at least eight glasses a day, and stay away from salty or high fat foods. I'd like to see a four-pound gain per month from this point on." He consulted the chart as he continued, to be sure he hit on every point needing to be addressed at the time.

"Have you and your husband come to any conclusion regarding the Amniocentesis?" He looked up from under his bifocals for a response. Her time allotment up, he interrupted Amanda's thoughts with another comment.

"If you do decide to have the procedure you need to make an appointment at the front desk as you leave. Just shy of thirty-five, the call is up to you." He closed the chart and although physically standing in the exam room, he was mentally somewhere else.

A little annoyed at his impatience, she spoke with confidence and directness. "My husband and I see no reason for such a procedure. When do I schedule for my next exam?"

EIGHTEEN

Six Months *Later*

The obstetrician looked pale and was searching for the right words, unconsciously warning Eric of the impending news. His body language was screaming behind his green gown and forced facade. Something was wrong and Eric sensed it even before he began to speak.

"Is everything all right?" Eric's heart began to race and his adrenaline pumped with fear. It was then that he noticed the blood droplets on the doctor's gown. Eric fixated on the red blotches and attempted to prepare himself for the worst.

"Your wife is resting now. She's fine." Eric couldn't help feeling guilty at his relief that a problem existed, but had nothing to do with Amanda. Nothing could compare to the love he had for Amanda.

Before the doctor had the chance to continue, Eric interrupted, "It's,..it's the baby, isn't it?" He asked this question with reluctance, knowing he would despise the reply. The time seemed to pass in slow motion as the weight settled upon his shoulders.

"Your son was born with a multitude of problems. I'm sorry." The doctor hardly blinked as he looked directly into Eric's eyes. "If I were to give you a prognosis at this time I would not expect him to make it through the night."

Eric swallowed, paused, and felt the tears welling. Emotions erupted and in a fog he stood and spoke in a monotone.

"Can I see my wife?"

"Of course."

The day seemed to last an eternity. Amanda, as well as Eric, was relieved that visiting hours were strictly enforced and what seemed like an endless succession of visitors had finally come to an end. Nobody had the right words nor could alleviate the devastating events of the day.

Room thirteen, located at the end of the hall, was equipped with a bathroom and lent itself to the utmost privacy and fabulous views of Mount Tamalpais— views wasted under the circumstances. It was quiet now as they faced, together, a tragedy of boundless enormity. Although the birth occurred over eight hours earlier, time seemed to have no bearing, as chaos seemed to travel in a flash. Amanda had been hysterical, immediately sedated, tied down and the intravenous lines had been left in to keep her fluids regulated. Eric felt helpless as he watched a mirror of pain reflecting back from Amanda's eyes.

Amanda's dinner tray was set by the bedside. The nurse checked her incision, adjusted her pillow and refilled the pitcher of water. She rounded the corner to exit and mentioned something about a note placed under the tray.

With dinner untouched and the comment going practically unnoticed, the two held hands and spoke quietly about the baby, trying all the while to push guilt aside. Eric hadn't left her side but once, to observe their baby through the glass windows of the intensive care unit. He leaned against the window, crying until a nurse witnessed him, distraught and glued to the window. She waved him in, had him wash, apply a mask and led him to the cradle that enclosed his imperfect infant. Eric touched the transparent skin of the tiny hand and looked into the eyes of this struggling being. Thankfully the infant who they had named Matthew was wrapped tightly, exposing only his albinism and his tiny head—an ailment referred to as microcephaly. Within minutes Eric was back at Amanda's bedside watching her travel in and out of her drug-induced sleep.

A nurse came to take the untouched dinner tray. It was then that Eric remembered something about a note.

"Can you leave that for now?"

The nurse, acknowledging his request, set the tray back down, asked Amanda if she could get her anything and went on her way.

Two hours later, after much pacing around the room, Eric worked on his makeshift bed. Propped in the bedside chair with a pillow wedged between his stiff neck and the wall with a blanket draped over his exhausted body, he made an honest attempt at sleep. He managed only to rest his eyes at short intervals between readjusting, due to lack of blood flow to his butt and lower extremities. The lights on the wall clock indicated a twenty-seven minute maximum rest on the worst night of his life to date. Finally, he stood, walked to the window and stared at the moonlit morning. He turned to look at his wife and again noticed the dinner tray at her bedside. He ambled toward it, uncovered the lid and, at first, saw nothing out of the ordinary. He carefully transported the tray over to the window to get a better view. It was then that he noticed a small folded piece of paper tucked partially under the plate. Careful not to arouse Amanda, he set the tray on the polished floor, picked up the note, opened it and read the barely legible scribblings.

The nurses told me of the tragic news. You have my deepest sympathy. I'm planning to give you two some time alone today. My shift starts tomorrow at noon. I'll be in to see you both before. I love you and believe an angel is watching over your little one. If there is anything I can do to help, don't hesitate to call.
All My Love,
Beatrice Clooney

Eric scanned the room for the near-empty box of tissue that he, Amanda and their visitors worked on exhausting yesterday. Amanda continued her drug-induced sleep. At six-thirty a nurse on the early morning rounds entered the room and rudely uncovered Amanda to check her stitches.

"Oh, you startled me!" Amanda managed poise and manners in every circumstance.

"Doctor's orders...I've got to check your incision and fluids. Sorry for waking you. "

Amanda noticed Eric who was standing by her side, eyes puffy and hair standing wildly in all directions, in dire need of a comb. He witnessed Amanda smile for the first time in twenty-four hours and was thrilled.

"Bad hair day, hon?" She pulled her hair up to emulate the disheveled mess.

Smiling back, Eric felt renewed hope inching between them. Eric reached for her and nuzzled his face next to hers.

"I'll be ready with my camera the morning after you try sleeping in a chair hardly fit for sitting!"

The nurse, still working below, took Eric's comment as a personal insult.

The defensive R.N. spoke as if she was quoting the manual. "We do recommend that spouses and friends sleep at home and therefore don't equip the room with extra sleeping quarters. We have to cut costs somewhere. Better there than patient care. My paycheck has been downsized to the point of humiliation, and you know...I really hate to picket. It takes me away..."

Her endless rambling ended upon the arrival of Eric's hysterics. The pain in Amanda's abdomen ceased her laughing almost immediately. Amanda forced a straight face, then lied to spare the nurse's feelings.

"He's not laughing at you. It's. . um. . a private joke between us. We can see your point, really." She strained her face to the point of pain.

The comment seemed to satisfy the disgruntled nurse. Amanda turned and caught eyes with Eric, whose face was bright red and ready to explode with more gut-wrenching laughter. He turned toward the window and took a few steps in that direction.

"How's our baby?" Eric heard Amanda's sweet voice ask.

Instantly his emotions switched gears to listen to the dreaded response.

"It's not good. We're surprised he's hung on this long." The nurse stopped what she was doing and seemed to really possess empathy. For this Eric and Amanda had respect.

"I want to hold Matthew before he dies." Amanda's tears began flowing. Eric reached for her hand and the nurse agreed to take her down to Pediatric Intensive Care Nursery. She left the room to round up a wheelchair.

Except for the swinging door from the nurse's recent departure, room thirteen fell silent. Eric, feeling utterly helpless, pulled the note from Nurse Clooney from his pocket and handed it to Amanda.

"She's such a good friend," Eric said as Amanda attempted to move her legs to the floor. "We are lucky to have so many good ones." He guided her body up as she planted her feet on the ground. Using her Lamaze breathing exercises, she was able to offset the pain. She stood at slightly more than ninety degrees, holding her stomach all the while, and ambled toward the bathroom.

Passing the nursery window they couldn't help but notice the dozen or so transparent cradles, each containing a swaddled infant in the hospital receiving blankets. Beneath were healthy babies. Most were sleeping and all were beautiful.

Consciously turning from them, they looked ahead to faced their own reality as the nurse wheeled Amanda, with Eric never letting go of her hand, into the intensive care unit. Two imperfect babies were housed in the unit; the other, so premature, must have weighed under three pounds. Passing first this tiny human, they approached their baby as the shock settled in a little deeper. In addition to the tubes and intravenous lines, their baby wore a diaper, exposing the grave deformations. Besides the white, practically transparent skin, the baby's head was undersized and malformed. The tiny face was odd looking. Matthew gasped for every breath.

Amanda gazed at her impaired, agonizing infant and fell in love. Her hands trembled as she reached in to touch her newborn. At that moment the baby opened his pink eyes and stared into his mother's.

"Can I hold him?" Tears streamed down Amanda's cheeks, touching the nurse and bringing emotion to her eyes as well. "There is a rocking chair in the corner." She motioned and handed Eric a receiving blanket with a squeeze of her hand and left the unit. Twenty-six minutes later the baby was dead.

NINETEEN

Eric, crumbling on the inside, played well the role of the less emotional sex. He walked beside Amanda as the nurse pushed her wheelchair out the front entrance of the hospital. The Saab, with the hatchback open, was parked in the patient loading zone. Eric hurried ahead to place Amanda's bag and a multitude of bouquets in the back. He turned, eager to help Amanda from the wheelchair to the passenger seat. Nobody spoke.

The ride home was painful and brought Amanda to tears for the third time on this dismal morning. Eric, prepared with tissue in his breast pocket, dabbed her puffy pink face. She took over when she noticed the car swerving into the other lane.

"Thanks Eric." Amanda hesitated then spoke again. "I don't feel right about leaving Matthew at the hospital. He was with me for nine months and now he's gone. I just want to hold him and keep him warm."

The comment touched him and a lump in his throat began to grow. He swallowed twice to maintain his composure. "Matthew's in a better place now. Just his body is left behind."

"Did you see how he looked at me when I rocked him?" Amanda's eyes sparkled with the single happy memory she and Matthew had shared.

"It was beautiful...just like you."

Amanda smiled as they pulled into their garage. The emptiness began to close in on both of them upon entrance to the condo. Somehow the home seemed to be too quiet. Amanda headed for the nearest seating which happened to be an over-stuffed couch. Eric helped her get situated with pillows and such and then began the task of making their misery somehow tolerable.

"How about some music?"

"O. K." He kissed her forehead and enthusiastically bounded toward the stereo. She couldn't help but laugh at his exaggerated gesture.

Eric turned his head but stayed kneeling, placing his CD selections in the changer as he spoke. "I have a surprise for you!"

The hit single from The Blues Travelers started up in the background. A tear dripped from the corner of her eye and soaked into the pillow she rested upon.

"How did I get so lucky?" She caught the next tear with the tissue she held in her hand.

Crawling back toward the couch Eric smiled. "What do you mean?" He beamed with pride and was hoping for some sort of a compliment.

"Lucky to have found you." She reached for an embrace and was met with more than she bargained for—Eric wedged in beside her where they cuddled.

"You've got that wrong. I'm the lucky one." He kissed the nape of her neck. She closed her eyes and felt at peace.

Nearly a week had passed since the birth then death of their son. The weight on Eric shoulders was substantial but he knew time would heal and the weight would eventually dissipate. Emotionally drained himself, Eric was challenged by the additional support required to help Amanda make it through the day. Each day brought with it hope and

the desire to feel better. Each day brought Eric and Amanda closer. Intimacy harbored

strength and power to move on with their lives.

TWENTY

The soft morning light reflected brilliantly upon the tiny casket propped, for now, above the earth. Visible through the arrangement of roses were the ornate marble carvings upon the casket. Craftsmanship that was sure to please the Almighty and the angels alike. The pile of dirt that had been unearthed for the burial stood waiting and, along with multiple headstones nearby, filled the backdrop with the finality of the moment to come.

A semicircle of loved ones developed behind Eric and Amanda. The pastor, who was also present at the church service, spoke of the better place the infant had found, and of eternal life for all. Eric, relieved that his baby no longer suffered and having faith that he, in fact, had found a better 'place', was dealing with his loss in a less emotional way than his wife. Amanda, for the past four days liked the feeling of numbness that Valium brought. Physically she began to heal. Emotionally she was unable to tackle her immense pain.

Nurse Clooney stood on one end of the gathering with a drenched handkerchief unworthy of soaking up another tear. She watched with sympathy the entire service. Standing behind Eric, to the best of her memory dating back to their wedding, was Eric's father. The distraught expression on his face was hard to miss. The wrinkles in his forehead had deepened from what she remembered of his face, and his eyes were bloodshot and, at the moment, dry.

At the conclusion of the service, Amanda added a single rose and cried aloud. Shaken by the display, some members of the crowd began to disperse while others hovered. Only family and close friends were welcome at the gathering afterwards. Eric, guiding his wife from the cemetery, was propped on one side while Gabrielle supported the other. As the rumbling of car engines rang loud in this peaceful place, the proceedings of 'follow the leader' began once again. Nurse Clooney was overjoyed to be included in this close-knit circle and followed closely the Mercedes that Eric's father drove.

The day was unusually clear as the cars headed up Wolfe Grade towards Gabrielle's. Nobody dared the driveway and instead made three, four and five point turns at the dead end and parked on the roadside below. Nurse Clooney was glad she had chosen her less fashionable but more comfortable shoes for the hike up the driveway.

She removed her lipstick and miniature compact from her purse and slipped them into her jacket pocket before heading up the hill. After opening the door for his wife, Eric's father locked his car with some electronic device that made a beeping noise. The timing coincided perfectly and the three tackled the driveway together.

Beatrice, feeling a little uncomfortable at the lack of conversation, reintroduced herself. "I'm sorry for your loss. I met you at the wedding; Beatrice Clooney." She reached and squeezed the hand she thought to be Eric's mother's.

"You must have us confused with Eric's parents. I'm Amanda's 'stepmother' and this is her father." The wife didn't turn as she spoke and her words were cold. Edward hardly acknowledged the conversation and luckily missed Nurse Clooney's reaction to the mix-up.

Beatrice wasn't sure if she felt out of breath from the shocking realization, now clear in her mind, or the constant uphill grade of the driveway. She purposely slowed to let Amanda's father and second wife forge ahead without her. The image at the cemetery was still so clear. The resemblance between Eric and Amanda's father was remarkable. Their jawline, eyes and build were one and the same. Surely, someone else must have noticed the similarities.

Since ceaseless sympathy was pouring from all directions

to the 'guests of honor,' and hardly knowing anyone else, Beatrice was at loss for words and found herself on a mission to feed her suspicions. It was just a hunch, but in less than an hour she drove on Highway 101 heading north. She exited at Freitas Parkway and parked behind the Bank of Marin. Checking to make sure the safe deposit key still existed inside a magnetized 'hide-a-key' holder in the glove compartment, she took a deep breath, back combed her hair to regain the pouf, headed toward the bank that housed a safety deposit box that hadn't been touched in almost a decade.

A recollection came to Beatrice as she entered the bank. She smiled as she recalled forgetting to remove the hidden key from the glove compartment of a car sold three weeks prior. The new, teenage owner must have thought she was crazy after listening to her concocted story about having to see the old 'clunker' one last time, secretly removing the key when the young boy wasn't paying attention to the middle-aged, eccentric woman.

"Hi, I'd like to have access to my safety deposit box." Beatrice appeared to the naked eye to be calm and cool, but she felt ready to explode and feared the worst as her hands shook inside her pockets. Small talk was not her forte at times like these, but she managed replies sufficient to fall into the 'chit-chat' category of the English language. The clerk led her past the vault and into a room the size of a small bedroom. The room had been virtually unchanged since the last time she was here to deposit her last will and testament almost a decade ago.

Rows and rows of small drawers filled the walls. Remembering approximately the location of her box, she took a step in that direction, checked the engraving on the key and scanned for box seventy-two. Finding it, Beatrice inserted her key while the clerk inserted its mate. She pulled the drawer completely out, picked it up and followed the clerk to a private room and was left alone. A small table acting as a banking 'butcher block' was placed at the center of the room. Setting the drawer on the table she began to shuffle through important paperwork and a few pieces of fine jewelry. In the bottom right corner was a yellowed paper with tattered corners. She knew the list of names was scribbled upon the scrap and a handful of vials confiscated from the trash at the Stanford Fertility Clinic would be in close proximity to the rear of the drawer. Beatrice realized she was a "pack-rat" and finding the vials after all these years only reinforced the self-knowledge. She took a deep breath, paused and unfolded the note. Brick Edwards' name jumped from the page, and as her eyes scrolled and heart pounded, Edward Black's flashed toward the bottom.

Feeling a little light-headed Beatrice pushed a utilitarian version of a bar stool under her behind and took the weight off her swollen feet. Carefully plucking each vial from the drawer then lining them up according to list order, she noticed residue in one of the vials.

The clock seemed to take her back thirty years to her "rookie" days at Stanford Fertility Clinic. Her heart continued to beat as it had that night, her palms, moisture-filled, like a first date. Her memory became fogless as the vision of the full vial came back to her like a revelation. The vial that contained the sperm sample was still saddled with a lid that apparently was not airtight. Residue adhered to the inner sides causing the foggy appearance on the vial, unlike the clear appearance of the others. She hesitated, turned the vial to check the label and noted Brick Edwards in faded black pen.

Facing the ugly reality of the circumstance, Beatrice hesitated, then deliberately repacked the evidence into the safety deposit box. She locked the box, gathered herself and left the bank. As she drove on automatic pilot, her thoughts of Amanda's father and his undeniable resemblance to Eric, were enough to make her ill.

The imperfect baby made sense to Nurse Clooney, but still she hoped there was an outside chance of mere coincidence. Saying anything at this point to Eric or Amanda was not only premature but extremely damaging. If they did share a father, they, in fact would be half sister and brother. What would become of them? What would happen if she were to become pregnant again?

Undoubtedly, Beatrice could count on sleeping for less than an hour that night. She was awakened by the worst nightmare of her life. Then she realized she was already awake.

TWENTY-ONE

Blessed with the attribute of 'fixer,' in reference to life's dilemmas,
Beatrice brainstormed for days, working on her plan of attack.
The route she decided upon used, not only her skills as a nurse,
but her access to the medical library. Each shift now was
concluded by an intense two-hour study on genetics in a back
alcove of the hospital's library.

So far, her friends and coworkers believed her research was
strictly confined to Rheumatoid Arthritis, an affliction within
her joints that had ailed her for years. In reality, homeopathy
had worked wonders for the pain and swelling of her acute
episodes, but the alibi seemed to satisfy everyone.

The information on genetics was vast. Living in California
seemed to lend itself to the latest breakthroughs with so
many studies being conducted in the UC system throughout
the Golden State. Genetic counseling was becoming more
common, especially among older parents stepping into
parenthood for the first time in their late thirties and forties.
Genetic counseling was also warranted for those couples
who had previously given birth to a baby with any genetic
abnormality. She sighed with relief, as she realized that another
deformed child would be highly unlikely. If Amanda's OB
neglected to recommend genetic counseling, Beatrice, armed
with the latest information, would convince Eric and Amanda
of its necessity.

It was only 7:00 P.M. in the quiet book-lined corridors.
The stale bagel topped with cream cheese sat partially beneath
the growing pile of notes, periodicals and texts. The large,
lukewarm coffee, laced with nonfat milk and saccharine, had

been nursed for the last hour and placed strategically for access without looking up.

Out of nowhere Beatrice was tapped on the shoulder. She hadn't heard any audible footsteps and the tap startled her. She turned to face the understated, shy librarian standing behind, to her left.

"I...I, really hate to bo...bother you Nurse Clooney, but I'll be leaving ju...just as soon as I finish some restocking in reference." Rita, the librarian, mousy and socially inept, was a whiz at accessing information. She could hold her own against the best. Beatrice considered her a 'little old lady' and was probably only ten years older. Her fragile frame ambled slowly, screaming low self-esteem, and her skin had 'pruned' prematurely. Right now, Rita felt she was imposing, which exacerbated her tendency to stutter.

"Oh, thank you, Rita. I always forget the library closes early on Fridays. Do I have time to make a few copies before I pack up?" Beatrice felt a pang of guilt as she took advantage of Rita, knowing full well she probably had no plans for the evening and would probably agree to staying all night if asked.

Tossing the coffee and bagel then adding new information to her briefcase, she left the library for home where she planned to compile and graph some of the statistical information for her genetic research.

The drive home was less than fifteen minutes, but felt like an hour as the long days began to take their toll. The daylight was finally turning to dusk with remnants of the day's heat blowing warm, but refreshing wind through her opened window. She resisted turning on her headlights until absolutely necessary.

Her message machine was rarely empty at the end of the day, but the volume of messages had decreased considerably since her daughter moved away three years ago. She found herself looking forward to the familiar beeping of her answering machine. Silence, upon entering her condo, filled her heart with loneliness on the rare occasion when no messages were left.

Tonight the machine was beeping. Gauging by the length of time it took to rewind the tape, there were at least three messages. The first was her daughter, wondering if she could babysit the following weekend. The next a hang up, and lastly a message from Amanda, wondering if she would like to join her and Eric for dinner at the local brewery. The thought of spending another night alone prevailed over her tired eyes and aching back. She walked into her tiny half bath, leaned over the basin, splashed water over her face, grabbed a hand towel and blotted as she picked up her cordless phone with the other hand and dialed the familiar number. When there was no answer she assumed they had already left.

The pungent aroma that filled the small brewery only added to the authenticity of the old time pub that it emulated. Rarely was there a vacant seat in the house and Amanda and Eric felt fortunate to be seated in one of the more comfortable, private booths situated on either side of the bar area. Amanda had insisted on waiting a few more minutes to order just in case Beatrice was on her way, and Eric reluctantly obliged.

"I'm going to have to ask the waitress to bring us another basket of chips before I pass out." Eric began the task of trying to make eye contact with the busy crew that ran the place.

"There's Beatrice, you can order that juicy burger you've been talking about." Amanda stood and waved Beatrice over.

Eric in the meantime had flagged another waitress who arrived at the table just ahead of Beatrice. After waiting for the initial embraces and for Beatrice to be seated, she pulled a pen and tablet from her apron pocket. "What can I get for you tonight?"

Beatrice quickly pulled Amanda's menu into her view and scanned. She couldn't help but see a resemblance between Eric and Edward, and wondered if she was merely stretching her imagination.

After they ordered the cholesterol-laden burgers, varying only in the sauce and preparation, their conversation began to flow freely. At Eric's request, the waitress brought Beatrice a chilled mug, foaming over with the Ale of the week.

"Thanks for thinking of me tonight." Beatrice's obvious sincerity made her loneliness all the more apparent.

"Well, our first night out since the baby had to include you." Amanda's eyes began to look glassy but she managed to sustain the tears that filled just behind.

"How are you two managing?" Beatrice hoisted the mug to her lips, letting the cold ale slide down her throat.

"Some days are harder than others, but I started back to work this weekend. I'm excited about a few projects I've recently bid." Amanda turned to confirm to Eric that the healing process was truly underway.

"We are even thinking about another child sometime in the near future. " Eric caressed Amanda with his eyes.

Amanda smiled then added, "We really want a child and have agreed to try again when the doctor feels it to be safe. He mentioned something about genetic counseling at my last visit. When that's through, I assume it's a go."

Nurse Clooney gathered all the self-control she could muster to sustain a casual expression, but was thrilled at the latitude she was given on the subject of her new expertise—genetic counseling. "Well, that's wonderful news, kids!"

Eric's tone grew serious as he spoke, the crease between his eyebrows deepening with concern. "Do you know much about genetic counseling?...The doctor slipped me a pamphlet at the hospital, but I haven't really..."

On the brink of eruption, she forced herself to tone down her latest factual extravaganza. Instead, Beatrice pulled some basic information from the wealth that she owned. "In nursing school, before you were born, the subject was hardly explored. Now, with people getting a later start on their families and the growth in medical technology in general, so much more is known and can be known, about the genetic make-up of one's offspring."

"Are you talking about amniocentesis?" Amanda listened intently to every word that was spoken.

"A common screening tool to explore the genetic make-up of an unborn child is Amniocentesis. Others involve tests on both parents before, or after, fertilization. Amniocentesis gives the parents the option to terminate a pregnancy only after a genetic disorder exists. "Blood screening and other, in depth, genetic tests prior to becoming pregnant give parents ammunition before a growing embryo exists. It's a wonderful science with a body of knowledge that seems to grow by the minute." She wanted to keep talking but purposely held back to respond only to the question, without turning the response into the lecture.

"Are you saying that we might have been able to find out ahead of time that our baby was im...imperfect if we had opted for the Amniocentesis or other forms of genetic testing?" The fright in his eyes was evident as the thought surfaced.

"Amniocentesis is an excellent screening tool. Many abnormalities are caught, but the pregnancy is usually in the fifth month by the time the procedure is performed." She paused, reached for her mug and added, "The decision to terminate a pregnancy when the baby is that far along is a tough one." The comment made them think.

"The death of our baby will always leave scars, but we still intend to start a family." Amanda scooted closer to Eric and leaned on his shoulder.

"You both know how I feel about needles, but I'm up for a few pokes if you're willing." He looked down at his lovely wife as he made clear his willingness to undergo the genetic tests.

Beatrice couldn't have been more pleased.

TWENTY-TWO

Four Months *Later*

The morning was cool and clear. The Bay was sparkling, reflecting the soft light of the morning. Soft music played as the Saab hummed through the tunnel that led to the Golden Gate. The steaming latte kept Amanda's hands warm and blood pumping. It was early and, by far, their favorite time of day.

"I'm so glad we don't have to deal with traffic today," she said. Kelsey, done smudging up the rear windows, nuzzled up to Amanda then licked her face several times. "And Kelsey is going to have a ball in Golden Gate Park. Did you remember the Frisbee?"

"She hasn't forgiven me since Yosemite. Since then it never leaves the trunk. I can't stand to look at that pouty face if I happen to forget her play toys." He too was soaking up the beauty of the morning. "Aren't you glad I asked if Doctor Goldstein had Saturday hours?"

"Four, no, five times you've been fishing for a compliment. Have my responses been unsatisfactory so far?...Oh, Eric, my love, let me kiss the ground that you walk on. For you, and only you, have dreamed up the perfect way to combine a genetic counseling appointment with a fun-filled afternoon!" Amanda giggled as she delivered her dramatic compliment. Kelsey wagged her tail, and her whole body, for that matter.

Eric, smiling, ran his hand over the dog's thick, rich fur. "Well, that's the kind of appreciation we like to hear, don't we, Kelsey.... Poochy Whoochy Woo?"

Their giddiness came to a halt, and even Kelsey sensed the growing tension as the car pulled into a compact space just in front of the austere cement building. Her tail stopped wagging and instead found refuge between her legs. The conversation abruptly ended as both Eric and Amanda had no words.

Leaving the windows partially open, Eric checked the address and turned off the engine. Amanda hoisted her backpack from the back seat, said good-bye to Kelsey, adjusted her bag and met Eric face to face.

"You know this appointment is optional." Eric stood facing his wife, placing his hand upon her shoulder and eyes upon hers.

"I want to know, even if it is bad news. I can't and won't allow a baby of ours to suffer again." She was strong and determined.

They turned up the cement path in the established Sunset District where they came to a sign that pointed them in the general direction of Suite 3B, Gerald Goldstein, M.D. The building, extremely modern to the point of being cold, was adorned with flowers and meticulously manicured shrubbery, making an attempt at warmth. Park benches were strategically placed for both privacy as well as aesthetics. With the exception of another couple enjoying their vantage point on the bench beside the rose garden, the place was vacant.

Inside, the fertility clinic opened to a small waiting room. Eight to ten chairs lined one wall, which faced the sliding glass windows that closed off the office housing the administrative staff. Four others clustered with an end table off to one side sat perpendicular to the lineup. Magazines filled a small shelf and brochures sat on the table.

Eric and Amanda arrived fifteen minutes ahead of schedule and witnessed the receptionist making an honest attempt to pull herself together. She attempted to hide the fact that she was applying lipstick and under-eye concealer instead of her usual duties. The young girl blushed as she realized she was caught 'red-handed.'

"Can I help you?" She stood, pushed her tousled hair behind her ears and leaned toward the opening in the window.

"We are the Edwards; here to see Doctor Goldstein at 9:00." Amanda appeared perfectly confident, but Eric could sense her nervousness.

"You're welcome to wait in here or in the garden out front. He's usually on time, but you have a few minutes if you'd like to take a stroll in the garden. If you turn right and continue on the path until it curves, just past the fountain, you'll reach the most spectacular vantage point in San Francisco." She seemed very friendly, but was trying to sell the outdoors, possibly to allow for uninterrupted make-up application. Optimistic that she was truthful, they were out the door to seek out the awesome view.

They passed the fountain and spotted the wood and brass bench as they rounded the bend. Established bougainvillea were climbing the trellises that formed a semicircle around the bench, giving patrons both privacy and wind resistance as they took in the sights.

"She wasn't exaggerating, was she?" Amanda was mesmerized as she took in the Golden Gate Bridge to her left, Fisherman's Wharf straight ahead and the Embarcadero to her right. The city's antique housing, painted in mostly pastels, filled the foreground and only added to the richness.

Eric sat next to Amanda and put his arm around her. "Only one other view that can top this!" He smiled and looked her up and down.

"Do men ever think about anything but sex?" Amanda cuddled and rested her head on his chest.

A few minutes later, the echo of footsteps from behind brought them back to reality. Turning, they saw a middle-aged man sporting a briefcase and gray ponytail. His pace was brisk and his expression intense. "That must be Goldstein." Eric looked at his watch; fifteen minutes had passed in a flash. They rose and reluctantly left the best view in San Francisco.

"His office is down the hall and to your right." Fully primped now, the receptionist motioned them through the waiting area to Doctor Goldstein's office. The hallway was lit with natural light from a panoramic window that occupied the length of the hall.

"I think this view is in direct competition with the 'bougainvillea bench.' Amanda spoke under her breath, paused, inhaled the view then caught up with Eric, who seemed to be a bit anxious about the time.

The office was decorated in loud colors and flaunted material extravagance. The square footage was more fitting for a suite and at first, before noticing the file cabinets, desk and basic office nook in the far corner, could easily be mistaken for one. The fuchsia carpeting and 'coordinating' mustard toned couch and loveseat, glared loudly from the room and stopped them in their tracks. The familiar sound of a blender was the only overshadowing noise above the opera music playing from the multiple speakers wired and hanging in various crevasses of the 'office.'

Emerging from behind a vinyl trimmed wet bar, the doctor appeared for the first time. Startled, but without losing his cool he spoke. "Please come in, you must be the Edwards." In what appeared to be a silver beer stein he sipped the frothy concoction as he walked toward, then met them in the entry way.

Eric reached out and was met with a wet, chilled hand. Amanda said hello as she eyed his drink.

"I'm Doctor Goldstein." He then went on to explain what he held in his hand. "It's my carbo-load 'smoothie.' Laced with vitamins, minerals and electrolytes; keeps me feeling young and alive. Mostly yogurt and fruit, but if I'm in need of a real jolt, I add wheat germ and broccoli. It seems to do the trick." Without self-consciousness or any apologies for his own eccentricities, he sincerely added. "I've got a few ounces left in the blender. Can I tempt you to have a taste?"

Amanda, open-minded when it came to the latest health foods, nodded and felt at ease with the doctor. She spoke for both Eric and herself. "As long as the broccoli and wheat germ are omitted, we'd love a sample."

"A couple with an open mind. I think we'll get along just fine." He set his stein on the designer coffee table, motioned them to sit on the couch and again walked out of view, with the deafening sound of the blender denoting his location, crouched behind the wet bar.

With tray in one hand, a rolling file cabinet in the other, Dr. Goldstein's attitude had deviated to down-to-business and serious. Setting the tray down on the coffee table, toward the file cabinet, he thumbed through a file, pulled it out and placed it on the table. Opening it first, he then reached in his breast pocket and retrieved a small calculator and pen. The pen, he put behind his ear, along with some stray bangs that grew from his receding hairline.

"I will start with a brief overview on the topic of genetics, then will need you to answer some questions. Please relax and... . " he pointed toward their 'smoothies', "don't be shy about slurping as we go along."

With perfect synchronization, Amanda and Eric sipped at their concoctions. Whether they liked it or not they both nodded with delight. Like Grandma waiting for approval on her holiday fruitcake, Goldstein was satisfied and continued. "As you both know, each human inevitably carries several...let's say...'faulty' genes. Rarely, however, do each of the two parents carry the same defective genes. Healthy genes from one parent frequently overshadow...or dominate the harmful effects of the 'faulty' genes. Your baby's deformities could all, or partially, have been genetic in nature. I suspect the outward signs of albinism and microcephaly were genetic. You two, in other words, have a similar 'faulty' gene or set of genes that would show up in all, or a percentage, of your offspring. Then again, your baby may be the result of an unfortunate fluke of nature that is seen on rare occasion in all species across the board. We also need to consider environmental factors as a possible contributor in the formation of your infant. I'm not talking about the well-known culprits like alcohol and second hand smoke. I'm referring to environmental factors that medical science has yet to uncover. The answer to these questions may never be answered, since an autopsy was never performed. Genetic counseling is simply a tool used to gain more information about your individual genetic codes, their relationship to one another and consequences for future offspring." He paused, let the information settle, took a gulp of his 'smoothie' then added, "Are you both clear where we are going with this?"

Thoroughly riveted, without needing to check with one another, they nodded and were both thoroughly engrossed in the consultation.

"Let's start with medical family histories. I refer to them as a pedigree. They're four pages long and very detailed. Do the best you can today, but you're welcome to bring them home if you'd like to discuss a particular aspect with other family members. With persistence, you'll be surprised what may come out of the woodwork.

"Let me give you some time before we discuss the histories. Following our discussion, I'll send you to the lab for a blood and skin test. The results should come back in two to three weeks. My office will contact you at that time and get you set up for another screening examination. Saturdays are fine, if you don't mind my 'smoothies'!"

He left them alone on the couch with the blank forms attached to clipboards and 'cruised' the internet at the computer on his desk in the far corner of the office. Twenty minutes later he returned to find that the histories were as complete as memory could uncloak.

"Before we discuss the histories, can I ask you more about albinism and microcephaly. Is there a strong likelihood of having another?" Amanda was afraid to hear Goldstein's response and felt responsible for the occurrence.

Goldstein understood the delicacy needed at a time like this and choose his words carefully. "I'll be able to tell you so much more after the blood work has been analyzed. For now, let me ask you both a question." His calm, confident manner reduced the tension and increased the trust. "Are there any known members of your family afflicted with albinism or pregnancies where the child was microcephalic?"

Before Amanda could 'fess up,' Goldstein continued his textbook discussion. "Albinism is the result of recessive genes; people that are carriers but without outward signs of the disease. Recessive genes work in strange ways. Sometimes they remain hidden for many generations waiting for two heterozygous individuals or carriers, without outward signs, to combine genetically. A homozygous baby or carrier with the particular disease can be born to these unsuspecting carriers which changes their lives significantly. They no longer take the creation of life for granted."

Amanda noticed a small window of opportunity and grabbed it. "There won't be any need to dig into the family wood piles. I remember my great aunt, or my great great...I thought she was ancient with all that white hair. I was young but will never forget her pale hair, pink eyes and practically transparent skin. I remember trembling at the thought of having to kiss the ghostly woman. I'll never forget the time, before my father had remarried. We were at a family reunion. I must have been four, maybe five at the time. She was there and I was terrified. I clung to my father's leg the entire evening. I was afraid I'd have to kiss her, and finally my father gave in to my pleading to go back to mommy." Amanda reflected as she spoke. "On the way home he told me that my Aunt was an accident in nature, but only her color was mixed up; everything else was completely normal."

Ashamed, Amanda looked down. "I should have told you after the baby was born. I'm sorry." She turned and was surprised to see Eric not angry.

The doctor was idle long enough. "Please don't blame yourself, Amanda. Albinism can only occur if both parents carry the recessive gene. You had no way of knowing this information before the birth of your baby. You are here now and we will attempt to unravel your genetic codes to ensure the safety and health of future offspring." The eccentric doctor hoped his words were soothing and clear before he continued. "I wasn't planning to delve into this topic today, and after the blood work is reviewed, we may need not venture, but recessive inheritance usually occurs when both parents are virtually unaffected by the disease. Unfortunately, they are carriers of the genetic flaw and can pass it to their children. Believe it or not, over nine hundred and forty diseases are known to be passed this way."

The man never came up for air, but was a wealth of information. "When both parents are carriers, each child runs a twenty-five percent risk of suffering from the disease. Another twenty-five percent would be genetically normal and unable to pass any flaw to their children. The remaining fifty percent would be carriers only, showing no outward signs." He smiled and looked his patients in the eye. "Even in the worst case scenario, the odds are with you, and early intervention can give you options, if the disease is passed."

Eric chimed in. "Do you mean Amniocentesis?"

"Amniocentesis is one method used, but can only be administered after the conclusion of the first trimester. If your fetus proves positive at this stage, the decision to terminate can be agonizing. Pre-implantation testing can be conducted at a much earlier date. Sometimes this option can eliminate the need to terminate a pregnancy if a healthy fetus is not conceived on the first or second try. These are just two of the many ways medical science has discovered to, one day, eliminate suffering of incurable diseases. Now Amanda...shall we start with your family history?

Kelsey was raring to go and, by the looks of things, had managed to fog each window to the point of zero visibility. What seemed like a blink of an eye had actually eaten up more than two hours. Mentally exhausted, Eric and Amanda decided to leave the car in the parking lot, squeeze a few of Kelsey's toys in the picnic basket and walk the few blocks to Golden Gate Park. The fog had lifted and had uncovered a crystal clear day. The sunlight warmed their faces as well as their outlook. Conversation was at a minimum, and for the first few minutes was focused on Kelsey who ventured in the street a number of times.

"Kelsey. . get back over here! You're going to get yourself killed." Hearing, but utilizing her selective listening skills, the canine took her time coming to her master's side, her mannerisms submissive and filled with hope that Eric would forgive her deviant behavior.

"I know it's exciting out here, you old mutt. Just hold

your horses. The park's only a few blocks away. Are we going to play frisbee?" Her favorite word was spoken, causing an instantaneous eruption of energy, exceeding the more than ample level that already existed.

"Get down." His voice was far from rash as he ran his hands roughly over her fur before physically removing her paws from his chest and tongue from his cheek.

Amanda lagged a few paces and was in her own world as they walked. Abstaining no longer, she pulled from her fanny pack a brochure she had picked up at the clinic. In her mind ran the statistics Dr. Goldstein had quoted regarding recessive genes. In bold print near the center of the page were the statistics resulting when only one parent was a carrier. Reinforcing Dr. Goldstein's words, once again, was proof of there being no chance of passing a recessive disease to a child. If only one parent carried the flaw, approximately half would be completely normal while the other half would be carriers only.

Was it all just a freak of nature, something in her environment or a huge coincidence that they carried the same 'bad' gene or genes? Anticipating the results of the blood work would be hell.

Day fifteen and still no call from Goldstein. After checking the answering machine for the third time, they forced themselves to run long in the evening. Mike had promised to take them on uncharted territory, which always led to an adventure.

The parking lot near Phoenix Lake was unusually empty for such a mild night. Mike's car was nowhere to be seen.

"What kind of leftovers can we zap when we get home?" Eric always had trouble holding off dinner, but had more trouble with sideaches if he nibbled anything so much as a small snack before a run.

"Either three-day-old Chinese or last night's pasta. I have washed vegetables if you can wait for the steamer." Amanda leaned forward and reached deep beneath her seat. "I think I recall a half-eaten Power Bar under here last time I checked."

"Believe it or not, a Power Bar sounds almost appetizing at the moment. At least it will fill the empty void without giving me a pain in my side."

"It's your lucky day...just a little Kelsey fur to contend with and you're on your way!" Amanda smiled as she handed over the hairy, half-eaten bar to Eric.

He bit into the bar, opened his car door and spit out a furry morsel.

"You really know how to turn a girl on!" She laughed.

"Someone's gotta keep the marriage alive!"

"Why is it I'm without a camera when I need it most?" Amanda turned from Eric at the sound of an engine.

"You'll be jealous when your blood sugar drops while mine continues to hold!"

Mike pulled into the unpaved parking lot. Amanda was already walking around to the driver's side while Eric toiled with stringing his ignition key onto his shoelace.

Mike, dressed in a suit and tie, bolted from the car with the Info-channel's latest dust mop. "Sorry I'm late. When the city council decides to get its priorities straight and pave the 'frigging' road, maybe I will exceed five miles an hour coming out here!" Moving with confident grace, he quickly wiped the dust from the flawless BMW.

Shaking her head Amanda commented, "Missed a spot."

Mike looked up to see if she was kidding. He smiled and realized how childish he was acting.

"Running in your suit tonight?" Eric couldn't resist the dig.

"It's only the disguise that seems to be throwing you, my dear friend. Since when do you judge a book by the cover?" He began to disrobe, only to expose a flashy pair of running shorts and a precisely matched muscle exposing tank. Slipping out of his work shoes, he crammed his D-width foot directly into his velcro-secured Asics.

Initially the trail was flat and covered in fragrant,

cushioning pine needles. Trees and other vegetation were dense and plentiful. Ferns surrounded the single-track trail as Mike led the way. Deer and small rodents watched and occasionally spooked as the runners passed deeper into the forest. The beauty surrounding them was astounding. Waterfalls burbled and drowned out their breathing. Conversation at this point went dead. All their senses were awakened; at no other time can a runner feel more alive.

Their pace was swift but nowhere near racing speed, allowing them to take in the sights. A mother deer and her two fawns drank from a creek less than twenty feet away. They stood like statues as the runners continued, farther yet into wildlife's territory.

Letting his mind leave the boundaries of reality and drift to a 'higher' place, a place that all runners seek, Eric felt he could run forever—or at least as long as the endorphins were plentiful. As much as Mike's quirks could wear on him, Eric realized the strong bond that had formed years ago. Their mutual admiration for the pleasures of the Earth bound their friendship together. Comprehension of the rhythm of stride belonged to a fraction of the population. This minority savored what the majority had missed. Eric, Amanda and Mike had all discovered a richness in life that linked the threesome.

Amanda held up the rear, only a few strides behind Eric. The baby had been born less than three months ago, and already she was up to snuff, with the exception of a few pounds of hormonal baggage. She found herself drifting in and out of thoughts surrounding work and her personal life.

The narrow trail curtailed conversation to infrequent comments on the land and exquisite terrain. Long silences among them were common, and instead of feeling uncomfortable at the lack of a topic, all enjoyed personal time to reflect, as well as dream about the past, present and future.

Only a year ago she dreamed of booties, the smell of baby powder, and the pleasure of strolling her baby in the midst of numerous admirers. Now, a nightmare replaced the dream and cast in the leading role an imperfect baby, dead and cold in his grave. Haunted for the past three months, Amanda found solace in running. She could attain positive ideas and constructive thinking, and could relinquish the nightmares, at least temporarily.

Occupying her mind at the moment was the breathtaking beauty, the magnificent curvature of Eric's legs and buttocks, as well as the rhythm of their breathing. Lurking in the wings, but without reaching the conscious level, was Goldstein's call. Every time the thought attempted to surface, the endorphins gave her the strength to override it and transport it to a deeper, less accessible, recess.

The ravine they were climbing seemed endless. Their breathing became deeper and audible. Less than a mile to the top, the three traversed Mount Tam's dense north side.

With much effort as Mike encouraged his tired comrades. "Less than ten minutes to go. Are you O.K., Amanda?" He glanced back to see her red face.

Out of breath she managed a reply, "I think I can make it."

"What, no concern for me?" Eric sarcastically remarked as he wiped the sweat from his brow.

The next ten minutes were grueling. The only incentive driving them forward was the reward at the top. Conquering such a feat includes so many inner rewards. Somehow reaching that point would make the pain all worthwhile.

A machete would have come in handy in the last hundred yards. The lush greenery was growing wildly and the path became narrow and especially steep. The momentum of running came to a halt. The terrain grew more treacherous, and they changed their gait to a swift walk.

A tunnel of light opened upon them as they crested the top. The view was spectacular and unobstructed for three hundred and sixty degrees. The redwoods and pines had thinned and the lush green grasses nearly reached their thighs. The breeze dried their sweat and cooled their bodies, and was harmonizing past their ears. The sun was beginning to dip and the sky was a blur of pinks swirled in blues. Their hearts and respiration returned to normal but their runner's high had fully settled upon their souls. With senses and spirits heightened they perched upon a huge boulder at the far north end of the hilltop. Sipping from their water jugs and feeling life to its fullest, they spent the next ten minutes in awe of the beauty that surrounded them.

The run back to the car, though harder on the knees, was restful compared to the trip up. They took it easy as the daylight left them, making visibility difficult under the dense canopy of trees. Reaching the car in less than half the time it took to reach the top, they refilled their jugs at the fountain and began replenishing lost fluids.

Feeling completely rejuvenated the couple said good-bye to Mike and headed home. Their anticipation grew as they neared the condo. They were lost in thought and said nothing to each other.

Amanda was disappointed that their answering machine wasn't beeping when they stepped into the living room. Heading straight for the shower, she disrobed, stepped into the glass enclosure, turned on the massage nozzle and pointed the jets on her back. She closed her eyes and let the heat penetrate. Following his wife into the shower, Eric crept behind her and embraced her naked body. She turned, opened her eyes and welcomed the nurturing. Holding each other, they caressed and made passionate love as they rinsed the layer of salt from their skin. When they were through they continued in the pleasure of holding each other and enjoyed their longest shower to date.

"Do you think we should call him tomorrow?" Amanda lifted her head from Eric's shoulder and looked up at his wet face.

"It's up to you, Amanda. It hasn't been three weeks yet, has it?"

"No, not yet. I'm just thinking he's a busy man and...I'm sure we aren't his only patients."

Turning the nozzle off, he slid the shower door open, reached for two towels on the shelf above the toilet and quickly closed the door. He unselfishly wrapped his wife, then himself. The telephone rang. They both sensed it was Goldstein, bolted toward the phone, scrambling over the bed to reach it. Then they paused.

"Let's let the machine pick up." Amanda was listening intently as Eric too waited for the fifth ring to occur.

"Hello, Dr. Goldstein here, I..."

Amanda clutched the phone in her right hand and brought it to her ear leaving her other hand to hold tightly to Eric's.

"Hello, Dr. Goldstein, this is Amanda." She could tell she sounded anxious, and cleared her throat, hoping for an improvement.

"I'm glad I caught you at home this evening. I usually wait or have the front office call during office hours. I looked at my calendar just after the results came in and noticed the approaching three-week timeframe we discussed at our meeting. I realize your anticipation under the circumstances and would like to meet with you and your husband as soon as possible." Giving no indication one way or another regarding the pending news, Goldstein paused ever so briefly for a response.

Covering the receiver in an attempt to muffle the sound, Amanda turned and spoke to the man straining to eavesdrop, laying on his stomach next to her.

"It's Dr. Goldstein...wants to meet as soon as possible. "

Mentally reviewing his schedule for the following day, Eric commented. "Anytime after two would work for me. "

"Three or four o'clock tomorrow or A.M. appointments on Saturday are available at the moment. Let me warn you, I've been feeling vitamin deficient, and made a pit stop at the health food store for broccoli and wheat germ. Prepare your palates and your bodies for a rejuvenating experience."

"We'll take the three o'clock, hold the wheat germ, broccoli on the side!" Amanda was pleased with her wit and felt much better as she and Goldstein both laughed out loud.

The ride into the city this time was more congested. Traffic was beginning to clog the northbound lanes. Luckily, heading south was less popular today. They cruised at speeds exceeding the limit the entire way. Eric's 'speed fetish' had existed long before Amanda met him, and unfortunately, in Amanda's eyes, had not been curtailed in the slightest, despite her persistent pleas. Eric placed the entire blame on the Saab's turbocharged engine, and never confessed to his obvious love of speed.

"I wonder what it would be like to go through the tunnel without that screeching sound drowning out the music." Realizing she was dealing with an unalterable behavior, she exaggerated her fear by bracing her left hand on the dash while she gripped the leather strap on the hood liner.

"Hensa," referring to his car, "has no other way of expressing herself!" His tone was serious, but the smirk on his face gave him away. "Besides, she likes the city and can't help getting a little out of control before the bridge. Cut her some slack, Amanda."

Eric possessed a talent at getting Amanda to laugh and lighten up, in situations where her expression was limited to a nervous stare. For this, considering all they had endured in the past, she was grateful.

Pulling up at two fifty-eight didn't allow time for revisiting the 'best view in San Francisco.' Instead they made a beeline for the reception area just inside the building. The room housed seven, excluding the receptionist. Except for a lone woman immersed in the New England Journal of Medicine, all were coupled and competing on the tension scale.

Tripping the entry buzzer, they watched seven heads turn in sync. Eric felt slightly self-conscious as he took a seat, quickly hiding behind a magazine. Unaware, or possibly not caring, Amanda waltzed straight for the receptionist to inform her of their arrival.

With the time right at three o'clock and the other patients scheduled either for later appointments or the lab, the receptionist instructed them to walk right on through to Doctor Goldstein's office.

The light in the hallway was soothing, but not enough to calm their raging anxiety. The office door was ajar so they entered without knocking. They ambled toward the couches and coffee table, where their 'smoothies' were awaiting their arrival.

"I guess these are for us." Amanda said under her breath as she scanned the huge office for the any sign of the eccentric man.

"My stomach is doing somersaults, but we can't hurt his feelings...can we?" Eric whispered then put his taste buds at risk and stomach up for rejection as he took in a small sip.

Swishing the conglomeration in his mouth, ensuring all tastebuds a chance at a rating, Eric was pleasantly surprised and gave off a signal of approval with his eyebrows. She raised her mug just as Doctor Goldstein appeared out of nowhere.

"Well, well, well.... I see you've already indulged in the best 'smoothies' west of the Mississippi!" Somehow the doctor managed once again to reduce the tension, at the same time sustaining the trust of his patients via his unusual manner.

Reclining in the loveseat, Dr. Goldstein seemed totally at ease as he looked at Amanda then over toward Eric. Taking a deep breath he began to speak from memory. His hands were empty of charts, graphs or medical information.

"The initial tests are complete. I want you to keep in mind that although we have a much clearer explanation regarding your baby's fatality, continuing the investigation of your genetic make-up, if you so desire, can supply you with a more complete picture than what we have available today." He cleared his throat and leaned toward them as he continued. They listened intently and hung on every word.

"Have either of you heard of Amaurotic Idiocy?" With the wealth of medical terminology at his hands, he had a hard time deciphering which were layman's terms and which were only found in physicians' vocabularies. He waited for Eric and Amanda's body language to answer his question.

"I didn't think it would be familiar..." He scratched his head, procrastinating before administering the bad news. "Amaurotic Idiocy can be described as a sad and fatal condition found in infants due to a defect in the chemistry of the brain cells, resulting in blindness, mental degeneration and early death. This disease is caused by a rare recessive gene, a gene that according to your blood analysis, you both possess." He looked down momentarily, then, gathering his compassion he raised his eyes and waited for the response.

Stunned, but expecting a blow, Eric reached over to hold Amanda's hand. "Are you saying we passed this Amaurotic gene to the baby?"

"That question can never be accurately answered because no blood was taken from the baby and no autopsy was performed to identify a specific genetic disorder. I can only tell you that a high probability exists, due to the fact that you two are carriers. Albinism is commonly coupled with Amaurotic Idiocy, giving my theory all the more weight."

"Not all our children will be afflicted with this disease?" Amanda's eyes were pooling, but she restrained herself from losing control and missing relevant information.

"Absolutely not. In fact, the odds of producing another child with the disease are twenty-five percent. Half will be carriers and another quarter completely clear of any genetic flaw. You see, the odds are with you.... " His pause instilled confidence and allowed the news to be fully absorbed before continuing.

"I would support the idea of future pregnancies. In your case, with the knowledge of your genetic backgrounds, I would definitely recommend testing, prior to the birth or implantation of any future children. I can administer a number of the tests and will refer out to only the best practicing physicians, when necessary. If you decide to have your obstetrician conduct the tests, or would like to see a referral list for second opinions, please feel free."

Digesting the news, relieved it wasn't worse, they turned to each other for answers. They were pleased at the greater odds on their side. They heard Goldstein out, asked a few pertinent questions, filled Eric's briefcase with the latest information, shook hands and were on their way.

Drained, but equipped with ammunition to insure a healthy pregnancy, they drove around the city in silence and eventually found their way to Golden Gate Park. Traffic was heavy and, rumblings began in their stomachs.

Amanda finally broke the silence as they passed 'The Hard Rock Cafe" on Van Ness. "I haven't seen the line that short in ages. Are you hungry?" Without waiting for his response, she began scanning for a parking place.

"I could go for a juicy burger, slathered in cheese and surrounded by a mountain of fries." Feeling fortunate, he spotted a parking spot on the other side of the street. He slowed, whipped an illegal U-turn and pulled into the spot with only his tail end in the red zone. All this and just two blocks from the restaurant.

"Besides, my cholesterol has been in need of a jolt. Since we've been married, I'm convinced all this low-fat eating is going to make me live too long! Sometimes a voice from within is screaming, 'where did all those triglycerides go'?"

Cracking a smile for the first time in hours, Amanda coaxed him to maneuver the Saab forward, hoping to avoid a parking ticket. "Left to your own devices, I seriously wonder if you'd make it to fifty."

Exiting the car then popping the trunk, Eric found a jacket, placed it gently over Amanda's shoulders. "A little meat and potatoes never hurt anybody!"

Cuddling under the jacket, feeling loved and secure, Amanda realized once again how fortunate she was to have Eric in her life. "I hope the Chicken Caesar is as good as it was last time."

"And the time before that, and don't forget the time before that...Gee, it must be hard to live your life on the edge, taking so many risks!"

She slapped his buns, then giggled like a school girl. Her melancholy mood had made a drastic shift for the better. She ran for fear of revenge; something she knew Eric would seek. After a fifty-yard dash, she took her place in line as the bystanders looked at the spectacle before their eyes. Eric, not far behind her, tripped but luckily caught himself before sprawling and most likely scraping off portions of his epidermis on the uneven city sidewalk. The people in line cheered.

Wanting to duck under Amanda's borrowed jacket, Eric attempted to minimize his embarrassment by acting cool, calm and collected as his red face returned to normal. "Even if it means a longer wait, my preference is a booth...hidden to the public, hopefully," Eric said under his breath.

"We may have to tip generously, but I'll bet they'll let us dine in the back office." She chuckled.

"You are so funny..." He squeezed her hard and kissed her on the forehead.

Within fifteen minutes they were seated in the far corner of the restaurant. They reviewed the menus, ordered, then waited as they sampled the french bread. A black cloud drifted overhead and the conversation died.

Amanda broke the silence. "Do we trust Goldstein, ride out more tests, or leave things as they are?"

The point blank approach caught Eric off guard as he was in the midst of administering a pat of butter to his third slice of french bread. He looked up for the first time except to place his order. He put down his food and faced the reality that a decision needed to be made.

"I trust him and don't think we need to look any further for answers. I just don't know if I want to become any 'chummier' than I already am with my genetic make-up." Eric paused, sorted his thoughts and spoke again. "As far as I'm concerned, I'm satisfied with the information we now hold. When we decide to have another baby, we can go through all the appropriate tests to ensure that it's healthy."

Surprised at his well thought-out response to her question, Amanda stared into the candle burning at their table. A few minutes lapsed until the waitress brought them their dinner. Not wanting to hold Eric away from his burger, she spoke. "I'm with you. It seems like overkill to go through any more tests at this point." The conversation was closed.

TWENTY-THREE

Three Months *Later*

Opening his eyes and realizing it wasn't a dream, brought the adrenaline flowing through his numb body. How long had he been lying at the bottom of the ravine? With consciousness came pain and the realization that he was definitely in need of medical attention. A double take at his wrist and the protruding bone made him really nervous. Other than cuts and bruises, and the goose eggs pulsating on his head, he could find no other serious wounds.

Slowly he propped himself up and inched his way over to a tree, where he leaned in pain. Brushing the debris from his body, he began to size up the circumstances. From the look of the sun, it had to be close to six o'clock, which meant he had been out for over an hour. Amanda would be arriving back from the airport soon and wonder why he was late. At least the note he left on the kitchen table mentioned he was running but unfortunately it failed to mention any specifics regarding where.

Bits and pieces of the scenario began to play in his mind. He had felt lousy from the start of his run. In fact, he seemed to be harboring a slight flu bug for the past three weeks. Forgetting his water hadn't helped matters. The dizzy spell felt, at first, like an earthquake. It was as if the earth was pulled out beneath him. He fought to keep his balance on the crest of the ravine. He left the conscious world soon after.

Using his good arm he removed his damp, soiled shirt

from his torso and carefully wrapped his ailing limb. Twice he moaned aloud, and the echoes ricocheted up the canyon as he toiled with his shirt and unbearable pain. Next, he propelled his back toward the tree, leaned into it and managed, with the aid in his left arm, to stand in one swift movement. Seeing stars, he placed his head down and crouched in hopes that he could prevent another unconscious episode.

Alone, taking what seemed like an eternity, he made the rugged trek back to the crest and back down to the trail head. It was there that he met up with Amanda. Panicked, she ran the distance between them and began to cry as she saw he was hurt.

"I've been looking everywhere for you. Are you hurt? Oh my God, are you trying to give me a heart attack?" She carefully kissed his face in areas not encumbered by wounds.

"I fell from the crest. I'm O.K...just need to have this arm looked at." The distorted appendage was visible through the wrap, and her expression showed immediate fear as her eyes focused on it.

Supporting Eric with her loving arms, she walked him back toward the car. "We'll take my car to the hospital." In a failed attempt to instill confidence in Eric and herself, she repeated, "You're going to be just fine," a number of times until Eric, through his weariness, turned, kissed his wife, and spoke in a sarcastic, but reassuring manner. "I made it this far without dying. I give myself a fifty/fifty once the doctors get their hands on me!"

"I'm headed for a nervous breakdown and you're joking. I guess it's true what they say about how opposites attract." She finally calmed down enough to find humor in his comment and for the first time in hours, released the tension in her jaw; a nervous habit adopted long before adulthood.

Pulling into the Emergency parking lot high on the hill behind the Marin General, Amanda couldn't help noticing the pale tone that Eric's face had taken. Setting the emergency brake, she exited the car, walked around the rear, opened the passenger door to find Eric looking up at her.

"It was like a near-death experience."

Compassion filled her expression upon hearing such a comment. She reached to help him out . "It must have been so lonely and terrifying to wake up at the bottom of the ravine."

"I'm not talking about the fall. It's the ride over I was referring to! Where did you learn to drive like that?"

"A comment like that warrants revenge. Lucky for you I have pity for wounded men. "

Smiling, they hobbled through the automated door at the entrance and headed straight for the reception area.

Eric was admitted at once after exposing the extensive damage to his arm. The nurse asked a few questions pertaining to his insurance coverage, then led them into a stark exam room where they waited. A meager twenty minutes passed, which they both agreed wasn't bad for an emergency room. Still, they were thankful that he wasn't bleeding to death.

A man in a white coat entered. Without acknowledging his patient, who was propped on the paper-covered table, he took some time to read the notes in his chart, summarizing Eric's injuries and the ever-so-prevalent health insurance information. Luckily, Amanda was equipped with his medical card, even though Eric thought it ridiculous and unnecessary for her to lug it in her purse at all times. Eric realized he could no longer poke fun at the unnecessary 'supplies' she carried, deeming her most prepared for any disaster that could arise.

Looking up from the chart, then placing it on a table beside the door, the doctor wiped the sweat from his brow before speaking. His voice was low and controlled, which somehow fit his dark pigment, masculine features and brawny musculature. A sheen of sweat was the only indicator that physical or mental stress had crossed his path.

"It must be a full moon tonight. The ER hasn't been this crazy since the fourth of July." He patted Eric's shoulder lightly and winked Amanda's way. "Hi, I'm Paul Whitney; you must be Eric."

Liking him already, Eric politely introduced Amanda then, on Dr. Whitney's inquiry, explained the scenario that led to the emergency room. The doctor, an avid runner himself, had recently run the same trail and knew exactly where the 'spill' had taken place.

"You definitely picked a poor place for a dizzy spell." The doctor carefully unwrapped the moist shirt from Eric's arm. "Didn't your mother ever teach you to walk slowly on cliff sides?" Eric felt fortunate that he had such a confident doctor with an excellent bedside manner.

"From the looks of it, all the cuts and bruises are minor. We'll have those patched up and as good as new in no time." He focused his attention on the break and Eric's loss of consciousness. "How long would you estimate you were out?" The creases of concern between his eyes grew deeper.

Eric sensed the shift to a more serious tone. He glanced at Amanda, who attempted a reassuring expression. "At least a half hour. . maybe closer to an hour."

"Have you experienced spells of this nature in the past?" The doctor was writing in the chart, but looked up for a response.

Eric, feeling guilty that he hadn't mentioned the frequency to Amanda, spoke to the doctor, knowing Amanda would need an explanation regarding his secrecy on the subject. "In the last month, they have really been getting intense.... the dizzy spells, I mean. At first I thought it had something to do with my lack of eating square meals, but even with good solid meals, the ground beneath my feet seems to move. I can't tell you how many times I was this close to yelling 'earthquake.' He raised his hand and depicted a close call with his index finger and thumb and turned to read the expression on Amanda's face, which surprisingly showed some anger dominated by concern.

"In addition to the dizziness, are there any other unusual symptoms that you've been experiencing in the last month or two?" Putting the chart down, the doctor carefully cleaned Eric's arm.

"I've been really tired lately, and my throat has been killing me for a couple weeks now." He put his hands on his neck. "I figured the fever meant I had the flu...maybe Strep. Sometimes

I can conquer these bugs with some light hill workouts." He paused, looking a little depressed. "But I can't seem to get a hold on it...Tonight was different. I felt like my old self, at least in the beginning."

Amanda chimed in, "Anybody who puts in long hours every week is tired, but keeping your ailments under lock and key is something I can't comprehend."

"I know I have been keeping long hours at the office, and with the minuscule amount of time we spend together these days, I refuse to put a damper on quality. On the few sacred hours I put aside for us on weekends, all I seem to do is lie around like a true couch potato. It's been so frustrating for me, Amanda. "

The doctor finished his note-taking, dotted the I's, crossed the T's. By the look on his face, he clearly had no intention of releasing Eric anytime soon. He exited to retrieve suturing materials for Eric's head and instructed the two to meet him in orthopedics where Eric's arm would be x-rayed, set and casted.

"I'm sorry, Eric." Amanda's compassion was evident in her eyes. "I've been too busy with work to notice how you've been feeling." He tried to say something, but before he could murmur a word, she continued. "The time we spend together on weekends is sacred. I've really enjoyed the lying around and snuggling. The mid- afternoon fires and hot chocolate are so relaxing. I miss the cool winter runs we've taken in the past; but I enjoy our relaxing time too." She paused before adding one last point to the conversation. "Not opening up to your wife about your physical well being is a completely different issue." She walked over to the exam table and caressed a non-wounded area, then leaned to kiss the less puffy side of his lower lip.

"I have no valid excuse for holding back information. After all, if I can't tell you, who can I tell?" He turned and continued. "If it's any consolation...I just didn't want to worry you for no reason, or bore you for that matter. I kept thinking it would go away like all bugs eventually do, if ignored for long enough. This bug is worse than the IRS. I'd like to shake it, but it has no intention of letting go!"

They walked down the corridor to the emergency orthopedics room. A robust nurse entered the room pushing a cart loaded with gauze, ointments, tape and plaster tools. Behind her walked Dr. Whitney, suturing materials in tow.

"This is Mave, the head nurse in the ER department as long as anyone can remember." He leaned in closer and whispered, still clearly within earshot of the old nurse, "Behave yourselves, or else!"

The doctor and the nurse worked in sync as Eric lay supine, concentrating on a crack in the ceiling that trailed to the center of the room where water stains existed. Even respiration took his mind away from the pain caused by the poking and prodding and ultimately the setting of his arm.

The doctor broke the silence . "Just out of curiosity, Eric, have you had any cold sores in your mouth in the last month?"

"Yes, but I really don't see a correlation between them and the flu. My secretary is always baking me nut-filled sweets. I've known for years about my sensitivity to nuts, but I have no will power when it comes to fresh-baked goodies." With his mobile arm Eric pulled his lip from his lower jaw and displayed the eruption on his lower gums.

"Any stomach pain or cramps?" The questioning was casual but Eric knew full well that the doctor suspected something specific.

"No more than one would expect from the bugs that are apparently having a field day in here." He gestured toward his abdomen.

"Well, that explains the heavy Di-gel usage this past month. I was beginning to think it was my cooking!" Amanda attempted to disguise the nervousness in her voice. Feeling famished and a bit shaken, she decided to take a trip to the cafeteria, giving the doctor and Eric some one on one. Mave finished up on the head wound and left while Dr. Whitney, satisfied with the set, began wrapping the arm in gauze. The two men were alone.

"I recommend you stay the night for observation purposes. You took a hard fall and should be happy you're still in one piece. The stay isn't mandatory and if you opt to leave, I'd like you back in the morning to run some tests. "

"Tests...what kind of tests? I'm fine." His tone sounded frightened but was coated with ample amounts of irritation.

Expecting the displeasure, the doctor spoke straight forwardly. "Dizziness is nothing to take lightly. Accompanied with exhaustion, the sore throat, mouth sores and stomach irritation, your symptoms warrant a thorough exam, which I have already ordered for tomorrow morning. The tests are primarily conducted to rule out possibilities." He paused and with a reassuring expression added, "It could very well be the flu or a stubborn virus."

Pulled from his denial for the first time in the last month, Eric sensed a feeling of relief that only a confrontation can bring. "O.K., I'll let my insurance decide. If they are willing to cover an overnight I'll..."

The doctor interrupted, "I had the hospital run a check. After a nominal co-payment, an overnight bed stay is one hundred percent covered. You've got yourself a great medical plan."

Amanda pushed open the door with her hip and carried a teetering hamburger and all the fixings on an orange cafeteria tray. Hearing nothing of the hospital stay, she was all smiles, exhibiting her cholesterol-bearing gift.

"You must be starving." She looked at the doctor and inquired, "Is the food as good as it looks?"

He scanned the tray. "Nothing to write home about, but from the looks of it, your choice will only cause minor indigestion."

The dawn's light began its journey through the crevices of the curtains, past the patient in the bed beside his, bringing rays of light that aroused Eric from a deep sleep. The wall clock situated overhead read six thirty-five. Amazed at how well he slept, after the initial snoring from his roommate and the ominous hospital sounds, he closed his eyes once again to be awakened nearly an hour later by Amanda's soft touch.

"Hey sleepy head." Her lips pressed against his was always Eric's favorite way to start the day. In the midst of the kiss came the full realization of his locale. Afraid of the unknown, he forced a smile and tried to think positive.

Breakfast smelled great and was served to his roommate and seemingly every other patient as well. Finally the nurse informed Eric he would need to hold off until the conclusion of his tests. Luckily, the hamburger continued to weigh heavy in the pit of his stomach and, although he found the aroma pleasing, eating was the farthest thought from his mind.

By ten A.M. every orifice of his body had been tampered with, enough blood had been taken to fill a water trough, and he gathered numerous nurses could accurately sketch his ass from memory. All in all the morning had been memorable to say the least. Amanda wheeled him from one end of the hospital to the other, leaving his side only when necessary, making him the luckiest man in the world.

Happy to discard the butt-exposing gown in the hamper, he dressed his bruised body in the sweats Amanda had neatly packed, then propped himself back on his bed where the lunch tray had been waiting. He devoured the unexpectedly delicious BLT and tasty soup in less than five minutes.

Doctor Whitney appeared for the first time today with chart in hand and encouragement on his face. "Good morning to you both." He removed the bandage on Eric's head to take a peek, "I hope the technicians weren't too hard on you this morning?"

"Only my dignity is wounded," Eric replied.

Knowing exactly what Eric was referring too, the doctor smiled. "You've seen one, you've seen them all...well, unless you have something extreme to display! Anyway, the Christmas parties would be dull without all the 'visual material' we compare and contrast." Amanda and Eric were doubled over on the bed, laughing from their guts, and at the same time amazed at how blatantly Whitney spoke.

"O.K., let's get down to business." His personality took a one-hundred-eighty-degree turnaround. "The tests are finished for today. We won't know anything conclusive for at least forty-eight hours. Take it easy for the next couple of days. I'll notify you as soon as I know anything."

Feeling rejuvenated from the energy contained in the hospital meal, Eric felt confident that the tests would all conclude that he was in perfect health. "I'm feeling great today, even after my blood was siphoned and is contained in small vials lining the shelves of your lab. If it wasn't for my arm, I'd be up in the mountains right now."

Turning toward Amanda the doctor spoke. "I know you'll see to it that he rests." Amanda could hear the seriousness in his voice.

"I have my ways."

Just as his body language spoke of the conclusion of today's visit, Doctor Whitney's name sounded through the paging system. "Doctor Whitney to the ER...Doctor Whitney to the ER."

"Well, I've authorized your checkout and will speak to you soon." Hardly waiting for acknowledgment, as harried mannerisms began surfacing, he turned and exited.

"Just one more thing..." Eric initially forced a straight face which eventually lost the battle with an ear-to-ear smile. "Since I've reached the ranks of a specimen, I'm relieved about last year's removal of an unsightly skin tag on my ass!"

"I wish you could have held out until after Christmas!"

TWENTY-FOUR

Two Months *Later*

The grim unit screamed "no nonsense" with the simplistic sturdy furniture and practically vacant wall space. Any length of time spent, in what patients refer to as the 'hole,' forced the deepest fears regarding death to the surface. The reception area was stripped of flowers, fish tanks, colorful prints or magazines. The only reading material available was a precarious stack of brochures on a pressed-wood coffee table in the center of the room. People, all fighting for their lives, filled the waiting area. Most were older, slouched from weakness and bald from treatments, terror darting behind their sunken eyes.

Eric sat in the only available chair while Amanda stood beside him. From his vantage point he could read the bold title on the brochures, making the moment more frightening somehow. "Chemotherapy and You" titled each brochure in a bold black font. Thank God Amanda had the gumption to pick one up before Eric was hailed for treatment. He sure the hell didn't.

At Eric's request, Amanda stayed put until he was situated in the Chemo-Unit. She used her time wisely and immersed herself in the information she retrieved from the medical library earlier in the week. Her analytical approach to Eric's illness, rather than emotional, was not only holding her together, but provided her with ammunition to aid Eric in his fight.

Walking into the death-infested hallway, he turned, winked her way and followed the emotionless nurse to the Chemo-

Unit. He was instructed to take a seat in a small lab where a meager amount of blood was taken and quickly analyzed for a white cell count. The sober nurse hardly spoke, which made him seriously wonder why anyone would choose a job in such a depressing field. He smiled to himself as he envisioned, "No Small Talk Allowed," spray painted on the wall across from the seating area. His smile faded as the thought continued. Why would anybody in their right mind partake in small talk with someone whose life expectancy is drastically shorter than their pet goldfish?

His blood pressure and temperature were read and charted before he stepped upon the high-tech scale located in the corner of the lab. A doctor, announcing the conclusion of the days preliminaries, brought the suspected news on his white cell count and led Eric into the adjacent room. He noticed the large room was divided into eight to ten curtained-off areas where the actual Chemo treatments were conducted. Eric, as instructed, lay on the noisy paper-covered table, adjusting himself in a futile attempt to find comfort on the sterile utilitarian device. Trying to stay focused and latch onto the positives in his life, he blurred his eyes toward the ceiling. The doctor left to wheel in a drip filled with anti-nausea medicine to start the fun-filled day.

It was then that Eric began to drift and encounter an out-of-body experience. He watched passively, from a bystander's perspective, as the doctor plunged a sizeable needle into a vein and connected a sack of medicine-laden fluid to a metal stand. Eric lay alone for a number a minutes until a nurse led Amanda to his curtained off cubicle.

Amanda noticed a strange smell coming from the Chemo-Unit even before entering. The quiet could be compared to the low rumble of a library. Her legs were unsteady and she began to feel lightheaded. Taking a deep breath she gathered her strength and forged ahead. Unfortunately, opened partitions along the way told stories of battles being fought alone. Nobody to hold their hand. This was almost unbearable, but seeing Eric lying there, so beautiful and strong, she was sure they could beat it. She would allow no negative thoughts to enter and strived to not lose her cool.

Forty-eight hours had elapsed since the treatment and still Eric lay, close to death itself, on the makeshift camp Amanda had set up on the bathroom floor. Not a moment passed without her soft hand stroking some area of his forlorn being, nor could he predict anything other than dry heaves reverberating from his insides. The warm washcloth rested on his forehead; a foam mattress made the tiles bearable. Pillows were nestled all around his 'bed', and with the slightest muscle moved, Amanda adjusted the pillows to aid in his comfort. Amanda's altruistic love warmed his soul, but true pleasure came with sleep and the remote possibility of dreams about life before leukemia.

Upon opening his eyes, he was again plagued with the harsh reality of the battle he was fighting. Eric was convinced that if the leukemia didn't claim his life, the massive doses of radiation and chemotherapy drugs would surely do the trick. Undertaking the treatments, the side effects prepared him for the agony he would undergo in months to come. Losing his hair in the next few weeks seemed less important. To keep him warm, or possibly get accustomed to his future 'look', Amanda had retrieved a "beanie" to cover his chilled and soon to be exposed head. The nausea suppositories seemed to be a waste of time, but Amanda insisted they couldn't hurt and made sure they were inserted like clockwork. Ice cubes caused the gag reflex but dehydration equated to driving back to the hospital, giving him the incentive needed to ingest meager amounts of fluid.

The doorbell rang. At first, Amanda had no intention of answering. The persistent caller continued ringing, forcing Amanda to at least look through the peephole. Quietly she crept to the door and saw Beatrice stacking boxes of sorts on the porch. Amanda unlocked and turned the knob. Her tired eyes were met with intense sympathy and a bolt of strength.

"I'm so sorry to intrude Amanda. I think I know what

you're going through and I want to help. I brought you some prepared meals to give you some time to rest. I guarantee his appetite will be in full force in a matter of days."

"I sure hope you're right. Keeping an ice cube down is a monumental feat these days. He already is looking gaunt."

"And so are you. When is the last time you've eaten, or slept for that matter?"

"I know, I know, but I think we are through the worst of it now." Amanda paused and her eyes watered. "I can't imagine him getting any worse."

"Why don't you get some sleep and I'll take over for awhile? I promise to go as soon as you wake up. You'll feel refreshed. Eric needs all your strength."

Feeling like a bit of a failure, Amanda agreed to let her stay for a short while. Anyhow, Amanda knew Beatrice was right. Amanda had handled her own affairs since she was a young girl and obliging to everyone's generosity was going to take some practice.

Three and a half hours later, Amanda rose from her slumber, showered and began dressing. She felt refreshed as she stood in front of the mirror to clip her hair back. Vapors were traveling swiftly from the kitchen and managed to fill the steamy bathroom with an aroma that caused her to salivate. In less than a minute she threw on some sweats and a coat of lipstick and was able to make it to the kitchen just as the hearty lasagna was served. Beatrice joined her with a cup a tea and intermittently checked on Eric. They hardly talked and Beatrice continued reading the book she brought along. The unspoken words were loud and clear as Beatrice had mastered non-verbal subtleties decades ago. She gave Amanda all the space she needed and looked up from her novel and commented. "I found I'm not as limber as I used to be. I sat on the floor for the first couple of hours and could swear my entire body had convulsed into one giant charlie horse." She was pleased she could bring a smile to Amanda's worried expression.

"I'm sorry for sleeping for so long."

"Sorry...don't be ridiculous. I don't have to be back at work until the day after tomorrow. I want to help."

"How can I ever thank you?" Amanda sat down next to Eric who looked no worse and possibly a little better.

"He was awake about an hour ago. I told him you were resting, which made him happy. We agreed that it was hard to tell who was the sick one, you or Eric. The rest has brought some color back to your cheeks." Beatrice paused. "I think he's over the hump." Beatrice knew, in the back of her mind, that she might be forced to divulge what she suspected about their biological relationship. Siblings are the likely candidates for donations in a bone marrow transplant. If the Chemo failed, Amanda's bone marrow might be his only hope. For now, she prayed for Eric's recovery and planned to do everything in her power to help her struggling friends.

Fourteen days later the fingerstick was all the blood they needed to check for the 'white' count. White cells aid the immune system and help to fend off illness. A healthy individual can expect a count somewhere in the five to ten thousand range. Eric was shooting for three thousand or what doctors refer to as the three point.

He was alone but planned to meet Amanda in the Chemo-Unit in an hour. They quarreled earlier but Eric held his ground about her continuing some life not related to him or his condition. Today, after severe coercion, she decided to indulge in a long trail run. He closed his eyes for a moment as he waited for his fingertip to be pricked. Briefly he escaped from the confines of the unit, its patrons and the death that surrounded him. In his imagination he joined Amanda in her run. He could feel the exhilaration as he roamed the trails without a care in the world.

The assault on his fingertip was a rude awakening back to reality. He opened his eyes and for the first time mustered enough strength to really look around. To his right was a couple who were scared out of their minds. The fear in their expressions, along with a full head of hair and ample amounts of body fat, denoted a first 'hit.' In their early forties, they stood out as young in the unit. To his left was a women, probably in her late fifties. Her transparent skin covered her bones and was left hanging in areas around her jawline. She wore a paisley scarf that was stylishly wrapped around her hairless head. Her eyes were recessed in her skull and it appeared that her struggle would be concluding soon, the look of apathy was her prevalent characteristic.

His people-watching extravaganza came to a dead halt as he was instructed to stand erect on the scale. That he was fifteen pounds lighter didn't surprise him, given the way his jeans were limply hanging from his hips. A few brief questions and comments were exchanged between the doctor and himself. The mouth sores and rash he had acquired as a side effect from Methotrexate, one of his main Chemo drugs, were his latest concerns. Hair loss was a given and was hardly touched upon in their discussion. The doctor did promise it would eventually grow back and it was the least of his worries.

He entered another vestibule in the unit which led him to the site of his second 'hit.' The setup was different. Still, a dozen or so curtained-off areas were provided, but this time privacy wasn't an issue. Instead, the seven or so afflicted individuals seemed to rely on strength in numbers. The curtains stood open and supportive conversation was in full swing. He followed nurse 'Personality,' as he later learned was her nickname, then sat in a lounge chair apparatus. The intravenous drip in the bag above each chair varied slightly, depending on reactions, sides effects, etc. The common denominator for all was the cell-killing agents contained in the fluids. Unfortunately, along with the fast-growing cancer cells, the drugs zapped the fast-growing cells of the hair and stomach lining, thus giving rise to dry heaves and hairless bodies.

Eric hardly was situated when an elderly man wearing the look of warmed-over death approached his chair.

"Hi, I'm Bob and this is Helen, Darren, Milly........ "

After the brief introductions Bob handed him a handful

of 'Saltines' and insisted that he eat them during the last five minutes of the drip. Nausea seemed the topic of choice and the 'Saltines' had apparently proven themselves in the battle against the worst side effect to killing cancer cells. Eric thanked Bob and was already in better spirits by the time Amanda arrived. The camaraderie amazed him and, for the moment, he was confident his chances of overtaking the 'grim reaper' had just increased.

"Hi hon." Amanda came with her smile, real or forced, and a duffle bag filled with the latest published periodicals, studies and information on Leukemia and other related topics. Setting down the bag that totaled nearly a third of her weight, she laid a big wet one, smack dab on his lips. Eric always admired her lack of self-consciousness but felt slightly inhibited in front of the crowd that existed.

Clueless about the observers who had tuned themselves to her every word, and truly frothing at the bit to expel something from her vast array of knowledge, she immediately dominated conversation in the unit.

"Hi Eric..."She leaned in to keep the conversation somewhat private. "Great news about your disease. USF has just concluded a long-term study on Leukemia and the findings are supporting a much higher percentage of survivors. Bone marrow transplants,...that is, if we have to, are far from hopeless, especially since you have male siblings." With the enthusiasm she brought, Eric no longer pondered the 'realness' of her smile.

"Do you ever come up for air?" Eric was inspired by her enthusiasm and he was sure he had become the instant envy in the unit. "I'd like you to meet some friends of mine." Bob was the only name he remembered, but Amanda was blessed with the social graces to both smooth things over and make Eric look good at the same time. The next hour consisted of dripping cell-killing medicines into his bloodstream, watching his wife at work passing out and recommending various 'literature', not to mention the ingestion of numerous 'Saltines.'

The next twenty-four hours were rough. Throwing up

every hour or so this time seemed like a walk in the park compared to his first 'hit.' Visions of 'Cream of Wheat' came much sooner than last time and fluids were staying put longer, holding hydration at acceptable levels, along with providing the flushing necessary to keep the kidneys, liver and bladder functioning and dispelling the Methotrexate. New to aggravate him were the slough of mouth sores that erupted on the third day of recuperation. He had been warned of the sores, but somehow he had felt he would be immune. Wrong once again, but he wasn't about to let the sores, nor the fact that his bald scalp never ceased pulsating with pain, burden his fight. On the up side, his sense of smell was heightened to the point that he felt like a blood hound. Eric would be awakened from a deep sleep every time Amanda chopped onions or garlic or prepared anything with pungent flavor or aroma. Fortunately, his appetite was in full swing by the fourth or fifth day and the heightened scents were a pleasure. Small, mildly seasoned meals many times a day seemed to help stabilize his weight without aggravating his plentiful sores. As long as he wasn't losing, he was satisfied.

A week had passed and Amanda was able to work from the makeshift office she set up in the guest room at home. Eric, feeling much better, was engrossed in several prospective treatments in the cure of Leukemia. A holistic approach, using visualization, meditation and medicinal herbs, was keeping his interest at the moment. Closing his eyes he began to visualize his white blood cells growing in strength and numbers. He focused and kept his respiration deep and steady.

Sitting 'Indian' style, with palms resting face-up on his inner thighs, Eric was deep in thought as Amanda walked to the kitchen to refill her coffee. Amanda stood frozen in the hallway, stunned and deeply touched at the sight of her husband trying something that she realized was stretching his conservative boundaries. She was thrilled that he had taken an interest in what he, up to this point, regarded as the "voodoo" approach to curing his ailment.

Opening his eyes, he smiled at Amanda's astonished expression. He opened his arms and waved her forward.

"I suppose you'll be expecting full credit for my recovery if this meditation has the healing power that it claims!" She cuddled and leaned into his chest. "Absolutely."

They were silent as they found comfort in each other's arms. Eric's eyes were at half mast when the thought finally erupted from her lips, rousing him back to full consciousness.

"Do you think we'll ever have kids?"

"Do you think the doctors were lying at the fertility clinic when they cited the statistics on artificial insemination?...Just because I'm sterile now doesn't mean those frozen sperm aren't gonna be raring to go when the time comes." Silence took over. "Yes, I think we will have children."

Reassured, Amanda lifted her head and looked up at the strongest man she'd ever known. "I needed to hear you say that again."

"Don't forget how I got my beginning." He cleared his throat and gathered his storytelling voice.

"I waited for years, frozen in a vial, surrounded by liquid nitrogen, until I had my chance with a egg! My owner had a vasectomy, but did I let that get in the way?. . No way. They thawed me out and I was as good as new...only more studley! I have all the confidence in the world that my pre-chemo sperm samples are just as raring to go as I once was!"

"I married such a humble man. "

Feeling both secure and content, Amanda rested back on his chest before she continued. "I guess a silver lining exists, even in the most horrifying circumstances."

Eric exaggerated his head movements as he scanned the walls. "I'm just looking at the walls to see where that comment came from."

"Isn't it all so amazing what we have found out about our families through this whole ordeal?"

"I know my father was only trying to make it easier by saying, 'Hey son, the circumstances were different thirty years ago, but I've been there, too."

"So you don't think your father had any intention of telling you where you were conceived, if the circumstances were different?"

"Let's just say...I don't think he would have ventured on that topic during half time."

"I guess you're right." Amanda reflected briefly then added, "In a way it's better this way."

What do you mean?"

"You know...with the genetic testing and all. Maybe the clinical setting would be better all the way around...you know, to really make sure everything is O.K." Amanda's sincerity was overriding her concern.

"What would I do without you?"

"For starters, you'd be forced to expand your thinking capacities!" she giggled, picked up a throw pillow and pressed it playfully against Eric's face.

TWENTY-FIVE

Two Months *Later*

The third hit had come and gone, as well as Bob from his support group at the unit. The death took its toll on the mortar that held them together, and when the despair was more than each could take, they carried on and kept each other from crumbling. Eric was near the conclusion of his second phase of treatment and, for a change, his white cell count had stabilized, making him a happy man. If it was possible to perfect the art of withstanding the horrors of chemotherapy, Eric had surely achieved this ranking. The second phase consisted of every other week visits to become 'one' with the diluted medications contained in the drip. Plenty of oral medication was prescribed and filled the 'drug' voids between visits.

His hands were terribly bruised from all the poking. From what he gathered, finding lines at the far-reaching extremities was standard procedure when one is poked as often as he. This precautionary, bothersome, not to mention painful measure was for the patient's own good in case of venous breakage.

Side effects, as well as medications, came in smaller doses now. The latest was strange feelings in his nose. Cytoxan, a new drug administered in the drip, was the culprit. Anything but vomit was a walk in the park. Eric's extreme lack of energy was an enormous obstacle at this point in the game. He tackled the annoyance with mind power, lots of rest and herbal remedies. The most recent bodily function to be altered was the lack of feeling in his fingers. "Strange but tolerable," he described the new oddity to the doctor.

Eric viewed life in much smaller increments, taking advantage of quality over quantity. He looked at life an hour at a time and found himself making the most of the limited 'up' time he was allotted. An hour of fun went a long way as he neared the conclusion of his second phase. Six months had elapsed since his diagnosis and the waiting game had just begun.

TWENTY-SIX

Six Months *Later*

Even the Christmas lights looked more brilliant than usual, and the spirit of Christmas had taken hold and brought him to the homeless shelter. Giving back to society had brought Eric unencumbered joy—and that he had no intention of giving up.

The last months had been a steady climb to full remission. He had much to be thankful for. His runs, initially weak and exhausting, had built up to levels near to what they had been before diagnosis. His hair had grown in and was cropped close to his head. His pale face had gained color and fullness. He considered life wonderful as he stuffed the packages out of view, into the hatchback of his Saab. He was running a little behind schedule due to an elderly Macy's employee who wrapped gifts at turtle speed. She was sweet, deliberate and took pride in her work. Thanks to her, he managed to spend an extra two hundred dollars while he waited. He was late to his much anticipated physical, but the fun he had on his gift buying extravaganza was worth it. His new lease on life would definitely boost the sluggish economy, he thought as he walked past the main reception area and headed straight for oncology.

Six months had come and gone like a flash. Today the hospital's blend of odors flooded his nostrils as Eric entered. The familiar watercolor display that lined the hallway had changed to oils. The old exhibit had been slightly melancholy, but this one was vibrant. His eye traveled to each piece with admiration growing as he neared the small familiar clinic. He jotted the artist's name on his appointment slip and made a mental note to inquire about the purchase of the talented woman's work. Only a short time ago, he took much for granted. Now he appreciated everything beautiful and good that touched his life. This, he knew, was the good that came out of leukemia. For this he knew he was a lucky man.

Passing the 'Unit', he deliberately kept his focus straight ahead. Today the memories hurt and the thought of ever having to return to the torture chamber made his skin crawl. He held his breath, but somehow the scent still managed to reach his nostrils. He turned back, entered the clinic with confidence and crossed his fingers. Nothing had changed, including nurse 'Personality' and the stark decor. The chemo pamphlets were scattered haphazardly about. Thankfully, the only other patient in the waiting area looked healthy like himself. Checking in, he took a seat just as his buddy, Mike, nervously entered the clinic. Eric, at first, thought something was wrong with Amanda, but Mike was quick to point out the loss of pay that he'd be incurring as well as his intentions of spending the remainder of the day with his best buddy.

"So,...this is where all the action is. " Mike reached to shake his best friend's hand. "I guess the fun will be well worth the retainer I opted to throw towards my associate. Besides, I can't remember the last time we spent the entire day together."

Eric was touched. "I see you wait until I'm well to relish in the quality time!"

"In sickness and in health applies to married couples only. Besides, do you have any recollections of the last few times I stopped by. Remember how I bored you to the point of full-blown sleep?" Mike's tone turned serious, "I just didn't know what to say to you or Amanda."

"Just to set the record straight, sleeping in the middle of our conversations had nothing to do with boredom. These drugs wipe you out." Eric paused then spoke in a whisper. "Even you would fall asleep at the Playboy mansion."

"I think you're stretching it, but I get the point."

Mike took a seat. The color had drained from his face.

"How do you deal with the suffocating smell in here? I feel like I could puke. Don't ask me to watch when they're extracting fluids."

"That's right...didn't you pass out at every immunization as a child?"

"Yes, and so far, my excuses for missing the blood drives at the office have worked."

"Should I call for smelling salts now, or get you a vomit dispenser?"

"Just give me a minute, I'll be fine."

"If only the women could see you now." Eric laughed out loud and was, believe it or not, in the best of spirits. "You've got to be the only living soul who despises hospitals and their paraphernalia worse than I do. Thanks for coming."

Mike lifted his head from between his knees and Eric could swear he saw tears.

The initial blood and bone marrow checks were concluded, leaving Mike and Eric with time to kill while the results were analyzed. No nurse, female lab technician or doctor was safe from Mike's probing eye as they headed toward the cafeteria. Mike had absolutely no pride as he gazed and drooled on anyone with double XX chromosomes. His eyes undressed innocent women and, remarkably, the reactions he received were mostly favorable. Somehow he got away with the sexist, vulgar behavior, which only reinforced, and made easier, his next voyeuristic conquest. Toting three new phone numbers into the cafeteria, Mike's mission was accomplished. Eric headed for the pay phone while Mike made a beeline for a spot in the cafeteria line.

"Amanda," Eric said into the receiver as he turned to watch Mike flirting with the hostess, "Mike's here with me.... Yes, I'm still waiting for the tests to come back...After we eat the results should be in...Yes, I remember how good the hamburgers are." He smiled. "I love you too...I'll call you as soon as I know...No, why don't you get some work done. Mike's planning to stay... Bye."

Putting nervous anticipation aside, Eric had no problem

devouring his juicy burger and fries. Skipping breakfast always made for a hearty appetite when lunch rolled around. He felt better than he had in years and was banking on the outcome of today's appointment.

Mike, on the other hand, was more interested in people watching than his lunch, but eventually was able to focus on his friend—after, of course, the bleached blonde in the booth next to them exited the cafeteria.

Slurping down his milkshake, Eric couldn't help but indulge his new obsession with his watch.

"Looking at your watch won't speed up time," Mike said. "In my mind, you have nothing to worry about; relax, and stop fidgeting."

"I can relax as easily as you can stop your roaming eye. You have five minutes to finish your shake." Eric pushed the timer on his watch.

"Well, at least promise me you won't feel the need to check the time before the buzzer goes off." Mike really enjoyed the harmless sarcasm. He waited for Eric to mumble a comeback!

Instead Eric sat patiently as the five minutes ticked by. He was through playing around. His face took on a somber expression.

Mike, picking up on the nonverbal subtlety, spoke. "I'm sure the doctors will sign you off with a clean bill of health. Hell, you look great. And...last weekend, at the race, well, you left me in the dust!" He paused. "No...if the leukemia was back you'd know it."

They left the cafeteria.

It all seemed to happen in slow motion. First, the news of the return of the cancer. It was deep in the marrow of his bones and would soon spread throughout his system. He had limited options if he wished to celebrate his next birthday. First, permission was needed from the hospital administration to go forward with a bone marrow transplant, a last resort as far as he knew. Second, Eric's permission to contact his brothers for a possible match was needed. Lastly, to help insure a match, he was strongly advised put his name on the National Bone Marrow Network as soon as possible.

It was happening too fast and Eric's movements and response to the questions asked were deliberate and controlled as the shock settled in to the dark recesses of his consciousness. Mike, dazed, just sat open-mouthed and repeated the words, "No, this couldn't be right." Eric, feeling the leukemia had, at worst, gone into remission, had the rug pulled out from under him. He had prepared himself for this outcome and somehow remained under control. He signed on the dotted line and okayed the use of experimental drugs. Immediate action was needed and, by the sound of it, his chances weren't great.

Wounded, the two men walked arm in arm, not caring about false perceptions or stares. They ambled down the long corridor that lead to the hospital exit.

A recollection came to Mike. "Remember when we were eight, maybe nine..., and I was convinced I could fly? I think we even had money on it. I jumped off the backstop. Man what a long way down! The cracking sound still rings clear in my mind."

"Worse than the pain in your broken leg was the fact that Jennifer Pearson witnessed the entire idiotic attempt. How can I forget the hordes of pheasant feathers taped on your arms. You've always been so stubborn!"

"I'll never forget how you acted as my human crutch all the way home. You told everyone my flying attempt was a dare, not a stupid kid who really thought he could fly."

Eric smiled as they reminisced. "Saving your ass,...Isn't that why I was put on this Earth?"

"This topic does have a point, if, for a minute, you could stop patting your self on the back, dick!"

Eric realized Mike was serious and responded by shutting up.

"Well, it's about time I carry you for a while." With the comment came a steady stream of tears. "Really, Eric, anything you need, anytime, I'll be here. I'm with you, and plan to help you fight this."

Touched, Eric fell silent.

Mike, friendly with the meter maid, had parked in the loading zone just outside the hospital doors, without a worry. Mike coaxed Eric to let him drive him home. "Come on, Eric. You're in no shape to drive. Let me drive you home and you can retrieve you car later. Better yet, the hospital is less than five miles from my condo. Give me your keys. I'll run here tonight and deliver it afterwards."

Eric hesitated, realized 'no' wasn't an option and surrendered to his friend's good intentions.

The local brewery was only a mile from the highway and, like a magnet, drew the two men to its door. Entering and heading straight for the bar, they couldn't help but notice the only other customers who were patronizing the place at 3:00 in the afternoon. The two seedy, rather buffed men with slicked-back hair, were chainsmoking cigarettes. It was obvious that barbells and weight resistance were not foreign to these tough-looking guys; their muscles rippled as they played a serious game of pool. Diverting their attention to the task at hand—getting plastered—Eric and Mike perched themselves at the bar and waited for the bartender to mix the whiskey sours Mike had ordered.

"Do you think I should call Amanda?" Eric turned to Mike for an answer.

"My cellular is right here. Just say the word when you're ready."

"Maybe I'll finish the drink first. I'm not ready to break the news yet."

"Good idea."

They tipped their drinks and swiveled their chairs to seek entertainment from the men now chalking their cues for a new game.

"Classy establishment you brought me to!" Eric spoke under his breath so as not to offend the bartender or the muscle-bound men in leather, who surely owned the "Harleys" parked out front.

"My first attempt at easing your pain, and you still complain. You are impossible to please!"

Several drinks later, nearly obliterated, Eric reached for the cellular in Mike's breast pocket.

"Whatcha doing...feeling me up?" Mike laughed out loud and gestured Eric to keep his hands to himself. The 'biker boys' will think we're faggots."

Eric became hysterical at the comment and practically fell off the stool. He regained his balance and what composure he could gather and slurred back. "They'll probably think we've been checking their asses out this whole time!"

Swiveling back toward the bar, Mike ordered another round. "Did you want my cellular?"

"I think it's about time I call her. She's got to be worried sick." Eric's expression grew sober, but the rest of his body language remained clumsy as he fumbled with the phone. Three times he dialed Amanda's home office number, only to contact the answering machine. Finally it occurred to him to check the time.

"Six thirty-nine!...She always lets the machine pick up after 6:00...How come you didn't tell me how late it was?"

"I wasn't aware of your curfew." Mike was unable to sustain a straight face and was outwardly pleased with the needling comment.

In a panic, Eric dialed his home number. Amanda picked up before the end of the first ring. "Hello?"

Clearing his voice in a futile attempt to mask his drunkenness, Eric spoke with lopsided enunciations. "It's...It's me, Eric."

"I've been worried sick. Where are you?"

"Club...something or other..."

Mike, eavesdropping, interrupted, "Eight Ball,...Club Eight Ball."

"Club Eight Ball." Eric repeated.

Silence. Finally Amanda spoke. "Isn't that the biker bar, low life...dive?

Eric's brain was slow to react to her accurate description and without thinking he responded, "Have you been here?"

"Actually, I was able to formulate my opinion by merely driving by. It didn't hurt to read about the occasional bar room brawl written up in the "Independent Journal." She allowed no time for Eric to respond. "Are you alone? Are you O.K.? I don't know if I should be mad or worried, or both."

"I'm with Mike. The leukemia is back. I'm not in remission like we thought." He blurted it out, knowing there was no easy way to break the news. No response from Amanda. Eric continued, "You have every right to be mad at me. I should have called you earlier." Eric started to sob, and for the first time they, not the Harley studs chalking their cue sticks, became the viewing attraction for the seedy crowd that had congregated since their arrival.

"We were so sure I'd beat it...somehow telling you makes it a stark reality." His voice began to crack. "You fought as hard as I did and to tell you is to begin your suffering again." His words were coherent but slurred and interrupted with tears.

Mike coaxed the receiver from his hands. Eric, too choked up to speak, willingly let him take over. "Mandy?"

"I'm here, Mike." She knew by the pet name, used only when the belligerency level hits a certain threshold, that Mike had also overindulged.

Mike wasn't suited for the caretaker position, but he was at least trying. "The news blew us both away." His enunciations had a lot to be desired, but still they out performed Eric's. "We thought a drink would somehow lessen the blow."

Amanda knew that Mike frequented bars often and the 'we' should be changed to 'I' in reference to whose idea it was to drown their sorrows. But under the circumstances she couldn't feel angry. Instead she handled the situation with kid gloves.

"I want to thank you for being with Eric. He needs a friend now, more than ever. I too, thought the battle was over. Why don't you two stay put? I'll be right there." She hung up before Mike had a chance to oppose her attendance in the less than classy establishment. Amanda had absolutely no intention of drowning her sorrows in alcohol, but knew neither were in any shape to get behind the wheel.

The news came as somewhat of a shock, but Beatrice knew a full remission after the second phase was statistically improbable. Still, her hopes were high and by looking at Eric she would have guessed he was clear of the disease. Bone marrow transplantation was the last resort. The dreaded moment was upon her, and the evidence linking Amanda's and Eric's biological past began to look more like fact. Amanda had called with the staggering news of Eric's need for a bone marrow transplant less than an hour ago. Since then, Beatrice had sat motionless, paralyzed by the news. Ethically, she needed to let her friends know about the fertility clinic that both their fathers used to store their sperm. Eric's father, Brick Edwards, had stored for future insemination after his vasectomy. Amanda's father, Edward Black, a struggling medical student looking for ways to support his daughter, donated sperm for monetary reasons. Eric's mother was inseminated with Amanda father's sperm. The seal was never removed from the vial marked Brick Edwards. The possibilities fast-forwarded through Beatrice's mind, as they hadn't stopped since her mistaken identity of Eric's father at the funeral. Could Edward Black possibly be the biological father of both her friends? What were the chances the names Edward Black and Brick Edwards were confused when the inseminations were conducted? Mix-ups happened everyday. Mix-ups of this magnitude could be catastrophic and the effects could last for generations.

Her thoughts were running rampant as she stared mesmerized at the crystals hanging from her valance. They twinkled and glistened as they refracted rainbow lights throughout her small living room. She called upon every mental resource she had to aid in the decision at hand.

Twenty minutes later she had settled upon a plan.

TWENTY-SEVEN

Two Months *Later*

The small coffee shop was shabby at best. It was Amanda's birthday, but since Beatrice had been taking double shifts to help put her nephew through college, convenience and low cost were priorities. The shop was located just two blocks from the hospital. By all means, Beatrice was determined to get Amanda, as well as herself, away from the hospital, for at least a couple of hours.

Amanda predictably ran a few minutes behind schedule, allowing Beatrice a casual stroll from work to the coffee shop. Beatrice intersected a sidewalk florist as planned, selected a bountiful bouquet filled with irises and baby's breath, surrounded by plenty of ferns.

Today was the day she planned to come clean with Amanda. Eric had exhausted all possibilities and it was time to tell all. Taking in the crisp fall air she cleansed her mind and assured herself she was doing the right thing.

She entered the drab eatery, sat herself by a window that faced a convalescent home and began to recite silently the words she had chosen to open the topic of biological fathers, sperm donations and bone marrow transplants. From a distance she could hear the noon bell chiming from St. Isabella's, a well-respected Catholic church known for its wonderful array of sounds. She checked her aged Timex and was thrilled at the perfect time it still kept.

The orange plastic seating was uncomfortable and sticky.

It coordinated perfectly with the beige, orange and brown decorative linoleum. Surprisingly, the floor looked new, as the style was early seventies. The grill was going full blast. Soon the line of customers would be wrapped around the building.

Amanda made her entrance, oblivious as usual to the heads turning her way.

Amanda embraced her companion, removed her jacket and leaned in to whisper something to Beatrice. "Let's keep the occasion under wraps. With these bags," she pointed to her eyes, "I'd like to be incognito today."

"The secret is safe with me." How ironic the comment sounds, Beatrice thought. "You look stunning, as usual, even with the dark circles." She too leaned in, then whispered, "Happy birthday."

"You are so thoughtful. With the shifts you've been covering, I'm honored to spend some time with you. Eric says you check on him every day and are even able to sneak him extra goodies from the cafeteria."

"I'm convinced that man has a hollow leg."

A harried redheaded waitress strutted to their table and interrupted the conversation with her voice not only a few decibels too loud, but sentences tattered with blatant double negatives. Ordering for both of them, Beatrice assured Amanda complete satisfaction.

"How is Eric holding up?" The waitress was gone and the subject had already been opened. Nurse Clooney figured she had no time to be inefficient with words disclosing her suspicions and therefore decided to cut to the chase.

The circles under Amanda's eyes, visible under the applied foundation, were noticeable at close distances. Beatrice figured she'd been surviving on less than four hours of sleep a night.

"Unfortunately the bad news came in on Tuesday. The news really disturbed us." Amanda's disappointment was apparent.

A puzzled expression came to Beatrice's face. The wrinkles in her lined forehead became deeper with the grooves between her eyebrows becoming the most tense, and therefore deepened.

"I was in yesterday, and Eric was sleeping. What news are you referring to?"

The words were difficult. Amanda's voice cracked as she tried to say them, "Eric's brothers, well...they were tested and found to be unsuitable donors. That brings us back to the drawing board. It's looking pretty dismal, to be honest. Emotionally, Eric is weakening. Hearing the news on Tuesday really has left him depressed."

"When was he admitted into the Laminar Flow Room?"

"It will be three weeks tomorrow, and still no good match.

"

"There's more than three weeks left in his sterile environment. That's plenty of time to find a suitable donor." The sweat beads began to glisten on her nose. Thankfully the waitress barged in at the exact moment, exposing her ample cleavage as she deposited a stainless steel teapot filled with Lipton's finest on the table. Beatrice took the opportunity to wipe the moisture from her face, clear the rehearsed dialogue from her mind and begin the history.

The first sentence came out smoothly as planned. "Things aren't as bleak as they seem." She reached for her young friend's hand and gave it a reassuring squeeze. She continued as Amanda listened intently. "I know of a possible donor, but before I tell you I'd like to precede it with a story."

Amanda was on the edge of her seat and had no idea where her dear friend could possibly be heading. She could only be uplifted at this point, but with past disappointments she decided to hear her out, before getting her hopes up.

The story of Beatrice's employment at the Stanford Fertility Clinic more than three decades ago was opened and ran through lunch and well into the next hour. Their Cobb salads were hardly touched and the crowd had dwindled tremendously. They sat, almost head to head, glued to the orange seating as Amanda hung on every word and Beatrice, careful to unfold the story in precise sequence, felt the weight of the secret lifting from her shoulders.

Everything was described in full detail. No corner went

unturned. The visual images that Beatrice managed to portray ran through Amanda's mind as if she was watching a movie.

Her employment, some of her coworkers, Doctor Welter, the whistling janitor, as well as a number of the patients who passed through, were described one by one and in full detail. Amanda had no clue where Beatrice was leading, or if she simply had wandered off on a tangent, but at this point she could probably draw an architectural draft of the clinic and summarize the way it was run. Amanda was in no hurry, and the conversation away from the hospital was refreshing.

The mention of Eric's parents coming to the clinic proved to Amanda that Beatrice was on to something. Amanda's lack of response bewildered Beatrice. "Eric's mother was artificially inseminated at the clinic." Still no look of shock on Amanda's face. She continued. "You see...Eric's father, as you know, was previously married and a vasectomy was performed after Eric's half brothers were born." Amanda didn't interrupt and was curious how long she'd been carrying information that she and Eric had known for less than a year. "His father was still young, and in cases like that the patients are recommended to give several sperm samples, just in case. His sperm was stored at the clinic, and luckily, for Eric's sake, was used to inseminated his mother."

Beatrice's words were strained as if she thought the news would somehow hurt. Amanda felt the need to relieve her and chimed in at this point in the conversation. She physically touched Beatrice's cheek as she spoke. "Don't worry, Beatrice. Eric's parents told us everything. Eric donated sperm before all the chemo. He was nervous and feeling really down. I think his father was trying to help when he filled him in on the details. Eric's fine with it and realizes medical science has come a long way since then. We feel confident that aided conception will happen one day for us, too." Hoping this would bring a sigh of relief to her dear friend, she continued, "So, you see, we already knew about the clinic and how Eric came into existence. We even joke about it."

Beatrice's face showed no relief as Amanda had expected

would be the reaction. Instead, she took a deep breath and continued closer to the conclusion of the story. The first sentence was a struggle to make comprehensible, but finally she was able to bring forth the shock of Amanda's life.

"Edward Black, a Stanford medical student, donated at the Stanford Fertility Clinic prior to, during, and shortly after, the Edwards were active patients. For many med-students, the monetary value of their 'sought after' sperm makes donating irresistible. He probably did it to help support you, as well as cover the exorbitant costs of schooling. Flyers are posted around Stanford's medical program buildings, to lure struggling med-students. A fraction donate purely out of egotistical fulfillment. Most, though, want to fill in where their meager paychecks, grants, loans and help from their families ends. Sperm banks, rather cryobanks are constantly enticing samples from intelligent folk, with med-students being their number-one target. They're young, usually quite healthy, and after the routine screening, all around perfect candidates."

Beatrice found herself sounding like a cheap sales rep for sperm banks. Amanda, leaving the conversation somewhere after the mention of her father's name, was clueless as to where Beatrice was heading. Her outward nervousness did show concern and for the first time, Amanda was afraid of the story's conclusion. A jolt of adrenaline raced through her body and clammy sweat emerged on the palms of her hands.

"At first, I thought there could be more than one Edward Black, so I asked you where and when your father graduated."

"I wondered why you took such an interest in him after the funeral. All those questions..." Amanda began to make some sense of Beatrice's odd behavior.

"After the baby was born and then recognizing Eric's parents at the funeral...the wheels started spinning."

Suspecting the grand finale, Amanda braced for the unknown. "What is it, Bea?" The fear in her voice complemented the terror in Beatrice's.

"Well, Marcia, the ditsy office manager at the fertility clinic who could hardly keep the files in order, doubled as a lab technician when other techs were overloaded. Her office skills had much to be desired; her lab skills proved to be hazardous, at best. I did a little investigating after hours one night...you know, to put my suspicions about her lab room inadequacies to rest." Beatrice paused, as if holding off the bad news would help to sustain the blow.

"And?" Amanda's arm movement indicated her need for Beatrice to get to the point.

"And...what I found that night in the lab was astounding. I was alone. Everything was in disarray, but surprisingly, everything checked out in the lab. It wasn't until I was leaving that something in the trash caught my eye."

Beatrice's eyes darted back and forth as if the clock had been placed back in time. She swallowed, eyes watering and faced flushed, "The janitor arrived at exactly that moment. I had one choice and quickly gathered the entire contents of the trash, liner and all. Locking myself in the bathroom, I sorted through everything, taking notes on pertinent information and storing, in my safe deposit box, the vials that I recovered." Reaching into her satchel that dangled from the back of her chair, Beatrice carefully extracted two tissue-covered vials. As she unwrapped them, Amanda sipped her lukewarm tea and braced herself for what seemed inevitable.

"These vials look exactly the same as they did thirty some odd years ago except for one thing." Beatrice positioned the vials as to display the faded but legible handwritten names inscribed on the labels. The first label read 'Black, Edward and the other 'Edwards, Brick, the names of her father and father-in-law. Amanda was afraid to ask, but did anyway. "What?"

Beatrice knew it was time to speak the words she'd been guarding for so long. "This vial," she placed the one marked 'Edwards, Brick' on Amanda's placement, "contained an unused sperm sample."

Taking a deep cleansing breath, she forced the hurtful words from her lips. "I believe human error was at play on the day Eric's mother was inseminated." Her words, practiced numerous times in front of the mirror, seemed to come out in slow motion. She could see that Amanda still was in the dark. "Don't you see, Amanda? Your father's and Brick Edwards' names are like mirror images of each other. Their vials could have been interchanged when the frozen sperm was extracted from the freezer."

"No!" Amanda cried.

"All these years I kept the vials in my safe deposit box. Why, I'm not sure. Call it a hunch about Doctor Welter and the loose way he ran such a delicate business. Never did I think my knowledge would lead to this." Tears streamed and collected in the deeper lines carved in her face. "I kept trying to prove myself wrong. The more information I gathered, the more I knew the worst to be true."

"So, you're saying that my father is also Eric's father?" Her voice was louder and wilder than she intended. Heads of other diners turned toward their table.

Scrambling to get her out in the fresh air, Beatrice gathered up their belongings and followed Amanda up and out the door. She never did get change for her 'twenty' and therefore left a sizeable tip. Nothing seemed to matter.

Beatrice, loaded to the gills with purses, her satchel and a beautiful bouquet of flowers, walked for a few blocks in complete silence. Amanda struggled with the enormity of the nightmare. Patiently, Beatrice waited for her to grasp the reality before mentioning that Amanda could very well be a donor for Eric.

Finally Amanda asked, "Did you quit your job after finding out how sloppy the clinic was run?"

Beatrice thought the question to be odd, but was thrilled that Amanda had broke the silence.

"You need to understand the fertility clinic was my first job after graduation. I lacked the confidence and the funds to walk out the door without turning back. Until I found another job, I stayed put and worked with my eyes wide open. Six long months passed before another came through."

"I can still envision the lab, as well as the rest of the office. To the unsuspecting eye, the piles of paper work in the front office and lab specimens lying around the counters may have appeared as work in progress. Anyone who frequented the place knew the disorganization was a constant. Small mistakes were made all the time. Fortunately, I'm aware of only one big one, but others are probable."

"How can you be so sure that my father donated sperm? Why didn't you tell anyone? There could be more than one Edward Black." Amanda pointed toward a bench that was situated near a school playground. Reaching the bench they both collapsed.

"After the funeral I couldn't help but give you the third degree. The baby had obvious genetic problems. And, after scanning my memory banks, I recognized your in-laws as the same Edwards at the fertility clinic. You must understand why I had to know where and when your father attended school and what he did for a living. Hearing that he attended Stanford as a med student during the time period in question solidified my suspicions and scared the hell out of me. You see, Amanda...until recently I had no solid proof of my suspicions." Beatrice deliberately paused, giving Amanda time to digest the incomprehensible before continuing.

"Still, I had to rule out coincidence. I contacted the Dean at Stanford. Within a couple of weeks, a thorough check of the archives revealed that only two Edward Blacks had ever attended Stanford. One a business major and one a medical student, attending precisely during the time in question."

Amanda and Beatrice were both mentally and physically exhausted. Amanda asked, "If all this is true...what am I supposed to do?" Her voice had a hopeless, depressed tone that Beatrice felt responsible for.

"Well..."Beatrice was surprised that the thought hadn't crossed Amanda's mind. "You could get your bone marrow checked out!"

The lights went on and so did the excitement. Amanda sprung from the bench then made an about face to Beatrice. "Are you saying...I could be a match for Eric?"

"It's a long shot, but if my theory is correct, you may be the only one to save his life." Beatrice stood and hugged her. Over Amanda's shoulder she noticed that the kids on the playground were giggling and pointing, but she didn't care.

TWENTY-EIGHT

"The bone marrow produces blood and is the third largest organ in the body. Acute Megakaryacystic Leukemia, AML, strikes the young and half of the afflicted die." The doctor, sitting directly across from Amanda, who yesterday extracted a blood sample for a possible tissue match, was obviously well-read, but he sounded more like an encyclopedia than a human being. She listened to him verbalize what she already had been studying for almost a year. It kept her mind from yesterday's needle, and did hit upon a few points that, until now, were uncharted territory for her. Obviously in love with the sound of his voice, the man rarely came up for air and continued his lecture.

"A bone marrow transplant is an extreme and dangerous way of curing leukemia as well as a host of hereditary diseases. The procedure has become more routine in the past eight to ten years, but the danger still exists. The diseased organ can be replaced by a suitable donor, usually a sibling. Same sex is usually a better match, but I have had numerous cases where opposite sex transplants were a success. If the patient is lucky enough to withstand the treatment, the next battle faced is the graft or replaced marrow. When the graft reacts against the patient, skin, liver and stomach problems will surface and mild to severe symptoms will appear. The afflictions may be chronic or acute, and they can kill. The greater genetic similarity between donor and recipient, the less likely the patient will suffer from what is referred to as graft versus host, or GVH. If the graft takes and the new marrow doesn't attack his cells, and if the infection doesn't win over the immune system, the recipient will live."

Amanda liked his positive yet clinical approach, but

she couldn't help anticipating the conclusion of his detailed description of all aspects leading to, during, and after a bone marrow transplant. The doctor was respected in his field and Amanda trusted every long-winded word he uttered. Still, enough was enough. Were she and Eric a match? Her worry about the answer began to block most of what he was outlining.

Amanda's blatant, non-verbal display of anticipation alerted the doctor to some of the more obvious of human subtleties. Focused on the wall behind him, she unconsciously tapped a persistent finger on the back of his desk. These cues eventually brought him to a summary, much sooner than expected.

He cleared his throat and changed subjects. "Your sample has been tissue typed and we have identified your human leukocyte antigen. The technicians as well as myself were baffled." He paused and Amanda was puzzled, wondering what her leukocyte antigen had done. "I called two of my colleagues in to look at the results. The match, although still preliminary, is much better than we anticipated."

Eyes welling over, Amanda spoke as he pulled a box of tissue from a desk drawer. "This is good news?"

"Surprisingly, the best—a match I can't begin to explain. I have never seen anything like this in all my years as a doctor." For the first time he smiled, which softened his face tremendously. "It was a long shot. Nurse Clooney wouldn't let up, and I'm glad she convinced me to try."

"Persistence isn't her only attribute. I love that woman like a mother."

"Of course, we'll need additional blood tests to further determine compatibility. The odds of this kind of match in two unrelated individuals is approximately two million to one." The doctor's left eyebrow flinched toward his forehead. Amanda knew what he was thinking.

Amanda entered the most sterile existence known to

mankind. She had been masked after dousing her skin with an antiseptic she could hardly pronounce. Fully suited up for her daily arrival at the Laminar Flow Room, she was ready to hear the good news the doctor had for Eric this morning. The room, 'anal' in every sense of the word, where Eric and his thoughts had been confined for nearly three weeks, couldn't have been more than a hundred and fifty immaculate square feet. Unfortunately neither of Eric's brothers were a match but ten days into his stay he was lucky to find a donor. The 'giving' individual, unfortunately, backed out with not so much a phone call or explanation. Eric's short-lived hope was crushed.

Struggling to keep his spirits up, he decided to wait the entire six-week period, the amount mandatory prior to transplantation, in hopes that a new donor would come through. With the odds against him, his counts plummeted by the day, making his other option, finding a donor, then starting at, 'day one' in the Laminar Flow Room, an excruciating thought that he refused to consider. Unfortunately, his HMO didn't share his point of view and stopped payment of the laminar flow facilities until a new donor was sought. As most would agree, life takes precedence over money. Eric opted for life.

The filtered air hummed into the small, stark room at uniform velocity. Eric's back was to Amanda as she entered, making it somehow easier for her to adapt emotionally, prior to eye contact. Beatrice had dropped the bomb less than a week ago. Today's appointment with the doctor confirmed the unfathomable. She held the facts to confront the truth. For a painful moment, Amanda watched as Eric washed his arms and torso with white washcloths. Each swipe warranted tossing the cloth into a nearby dispenser then pulling a new one from the stack on his bed. This ritual, using approximately twenty washcloths, occurred four times a day. In addition to the wipedown, antifungal cream was used in all the body's crevices. Terrible-tasting antibiotic mouthwashes were swished in the mouth on a regular basis. Only after six weeks of this body cleansing regime is the patient deemed ready to undergo the bone marrow transplant.

She had every intention of being there for the good news. She knew Eric would be ecstatic at a new donor being found, and convinced the apprehensive doctor to postpone disclosing information about the donor until he regained the strength to withstand news of that magnitude. With a desire to steer clear of a sticky situation, the doctor agreed to wait. With not so much as a twist of his arm, he concurred that Eric, in his weakened state, shouldn't be bothered with the fact that his wife happened to have a genetic make-up frightfully similar to his own. He happily agreed to keep the donor anonymous.

Eventually, after Eric had undergone the transplant and was making strides toward recovery, Amanda intended to tell him all of their past and questionable future. Her decision to keep the donor under wraps for the time being was seconded by Beatrice, making it a sealed conviction and the right thing to do.

How do you tell someone they accidentally married their big sister? Her thoughts ran rampant as she watched his emaciated but still muscular back pivot with each swipe. Somehow she felt incestuous and dirty and almost vomited on the spot. Swallowing hard, she managed instead to clear her throat and speak to her husband and half-brother.

"Good morning, Eric."

"Hi, Amanda, I was hoping you'd come early today. I sensed some optimism from the doc last night. Call it a hunch, but I think there's been a breakthrough. I'm trying not to get my hopes up...but..."

The doctor made his entrance and interrupted Eric's train of thought. In full Laminar attire, minus only the mask, 'Dr. Encyclopedia' had obviously figured the genetic coincidence to be an impossibility. At best, he must figure them to be first cousins. Amanda was hoping his subtle signs of suspicion weren't visible to Eric, through the doctor's professional facade. The doctor came with a smile and because of this Eric was bursting and hopefully oblivious to anything but that. Good news, a rarity in the field, must make moments like these worthwhile to a doctor who watches a large percentage of his patients die.

He fussed with his mask as Eric reached for his robe. "I've come to inform you of your appointment that will fall exactly four weeks from tomorrow!" The doctor was bubbling over and appeared to be warming up as an actor, his eyes moving carefully to Amanda then back again to his patient. He reached out to shake Eric's hand in congratulations and was instead met with an enormous bear hug.

"I knew it. . I knew it,...a donor came through. Whoa!" Eric's voice carried through the entire wing. He lurched at Amanda and twirled her around the room. Under the circumstances his strength was amazing. She appeared to be crying out of happiness as she held tight around his neck. She knew, and the doctor could see, happiness wasn't the only emotion at play. Eric had a fair chance at life and for that she was grateful. He never asked about the donor.

TWENTY-NINE

One Month *Later*

It was another morning and with that came the fight to motivate
herself to start the day. She sat in her robe, curled in her
bedroom chair next to a cold cup of coffee. Resting her head
on her knees that were pulled in tight, she caught a cockeyed
view of Marin's picturesque landscapes. The nightmares, with
the worst revolving around incest, recurred nightly, playing
back Eric's adverse reaction to the news of their shared father.
The most vivid part of the nightmare was his reaction. It played
out exactly the same each haunting time. Eric screams, 'liar'
and runs away. Amanda is awakened each time by her own
screaming, her pillow wet from tears.

For the past three weeks reality occupied her mind by
night, making the days less bearable in her jaded state. She had
shed several pounds and people were starting to notice. Their
family and friends attributed it to Eric's condition and the fact
that the transplant would take place tomorrow. All except for
Beatrice.

The granite counters in their small condo were crowded
with casserole dishes, most labeled and all washed and stacked
upon one another to make some attempt at organization. Half-
eaten pies and other tempting baked goods were displayed
haphazardly on the butcher block that sat in the middle of
the kitchen. Counter space was severely limited. The freezer
was packed tighter than a three-hundred-pounder in Spandex;
there was enough food to feed a family of five for a month.

Amanda appreciated the warm gestures from all who attempted
to express their sympathy. She had been taking the overflow to
a homeless shelter for nearly a month. All this food and no
appetite to go with it.

The doorbell rang. She opened it to the familiar lined face
of Beatrice. Beatrice brought her magnetizing smile and, like
all the others who visited, toted a vast array of edibles. Like her
own mother, Beatrice brought a tuna casserole. Before today,
Amanda would have sworn that the recipe died along with the
beehive hairdo.

The homeless will love it, Amanda thought as Beatrice
escorted her to the kitchen then coerced her into indulging in a
heaping portion. Beatrice joined her, adding to her plate a lavish
sampling of the other delectable selections. She poured coffee
for each of them and initiated a conversation. Amanda listened
as she moved the casserole around on her plate.

"What's going on, dear? Two days, and you haven't returned
my calls?" Beatrice too looked haggard from sleep deprivation.

"When I'm not at the hospital or attempting to hold on to
clients who are ready to throw in the towel, I find hibernating
the pastime of choice." Amanda's voice was lifeless.

"I can't begin to tell you how responsible I feel for your
state of mind. I'm sorry for barging in like this...I want to
help."

"You are the only reason Eric has a chance at life. Don't
ever think you've made a mistake by telling me." She reached
out for her friend and confidante and they both began to weep.

"Have you told anybody?"

"Absolutely not. Of course, I have to deal with the awkward
stares and whispering behind my back at the hospital, but to
them it's gossip and they have no proof. I hold my head high,
and as long as Eric pulls through, I'll never have to deal with
them again."

"But you do have to deal with yourself."

"I know. . that explains the depression, I guess." A long
silence took over until Amanda was able to gather some
thoughts. "What am I supposed to do when Eric gets home?

Should I break the news as soon as he's strong enough to handle it? When and how will I deliver the truth about us? Maybe I should vanish one day without explanation. At least I'd be sparing him from the harsh reality."

"Stop the negative thinking. You must go on living just as you were before leukemia. You and Eric are perfect together." Beatrice glanced around the food-laden kitchen, spotted her oversized satchel sitting on the tile floor beside the butcher block, retrieved it and rejoined Amanda at the dinette table. "I think I have some information that may help you change your perspective." She was all smiles as she fumbled through the massive bag that could double as a weekend suitcase.

"I hope you plan to pull a miracle out of there."

"No, just some facts. Food for thought, if you will." Beatrice cleared her voice, placed her dangling glasses low on her nose and began to read the computer printout. "Let me begin by stating that you are not alone." Amanda could see that ample time had gone into this research; there were highlighted paragraphs and footnotes galore. "For many thousands of years, marrying one's cousin was considered normal and common practice among tribes and small villages. We are all, in effect, inbred to a certain extent." Her well-rehearsed slant on the circumstances sounded like the opening of a documentary. It grabbed Amanda's attention as she took in every word of hope.

"In many areas of the world the practice has never been abandoned. In fact, consanguineous—"

"Consang...whateous?" Amanda interrupted.

"Consanguineous—marrying a close relative. Anyway, these kinds of marriages, in parts of Asia an Africa, account for between twenty to fifty-five percent of all unions. Fifty-five percent of marriages among Pakistanis are between first cousins."

"This is a developed country, the United States,...twenty-first century." Amanda found the stats interesting but still couldn't see how they were applicable to her.

"I realize that dear, and the practice is rarely seen here in the U.S. but we can't discount the religious and ethnic communities such as the Amish, Mormons and a group of people known as the Hullerities who sometimes intermarry. Immigrants from developing countries still practice close kin marriages, even after they've settled in the United States."

"I know you're trying to help, but—"

"I realize you don't fit, by a long shot, into any of these categories. What I want you to realize is that intermarriages are still practiced to some degree, in certain sectors of society." She paused, allowing her strategic closing argument, full of justification and acceptance, penetrate before the addition of one last slant. "There is no doubt in my mind that, had you known about your biological relationship ahead of time, you and Eric would never have gotten married. What you need to consider now is the love you have for one another and whether or not you can live with and accept the knowledge you now have."

Amanda sipped her coffee then mulled around in the casserole she had yet to sample. "Are you saying you support my marriage to my half-brother?"

Hearing Amanda verbalize, for the first time, the lowest common denominator, sounded harsh to them both. Stunned, Beatrice replied, "You love him, he loves you...what difference does it make at this point? We are the only two people on the planet who ever have to know."

THIRTY

Most had arrived at the hospital near the expected conclusion of Eric's bone marrow transplant. None realized the actual conclusion would take an additional three hours. Packed in the designated waiting area, Eric's and Amanda's families and friends were forced to make small talk, or at least some acknowledgment of prior acquaintance, either at the wedding or some other occasion relating to Eric or Amanda. Coffee and Kleenex were well used commodities, with speech murmured at a minimum.

One by one they filtered out from the stifling warm, tense surroundings and were led to the intensive care recovery. Each was allotted five minutes maximum. The nurse evaluated Eric each time before the next visitor was given the green light. Amanda was first to follow the tired nurse down the long corridor, through several double doors marked 'No Admittance Without Medical Accompaniment.' She entered a small chamber that led to the intensive care unit. Cellophane-covered blue garments hung from a closet hook. She was instructed to suit up, in a uniform similar to that required in the Laminar room. Any foreign bodies were trapped within her mask and gloves, away from Eric, who was not strong enough to fight the weakest infection.

A doctor entered the tight quarters to inform them that the operation had been a success. A sigh of relief came over all who were left behind in the waiting are; Mona, for the first time was able to take a seat. She kept to herself most of the time; Gabrielle and Amanda were the only people she cared to converse with. Hoping it wasn't too obvious, but not particularly concerned if it was, she clasped her hands together, closed her eyes and begged the 'Almighty' for Eric's survival. To her left was Beatrice, outspoken and down-right abrasive by Mona's standards. Undaunted compared to the rest, Beatrice tried to comfort the crowd by painting them a clear picture of what was physically happening to Eric. The blow-by-blow, though comforting to a nurse, was more than the rest could stomach.

Gabrielle, trying so hard to lend support to her only child throughout the entire ordeal, had worn down through the months, eliminating a strong shoulder and instead only having emotional instability to offer. Amanda never resented this, realizing she was doing her best. Eric's parents, keeping to themselves, hovered in the corner, went through a box of tissues between the two of them and were visibly shaken. His half brothers didn't show.

Amanda's father made his appearance for an hour of so. The sight of 'the biological father' made her skin crawl. She avoided him altogether, using distress as her alibi. Gabrielle, sensing her daughter's torment, managed to distract him and defer his attention.

Pacing in and around the waiting room was Mike, struggling unsuccessfully to keep his emotions intact. Sally had managed a little conversation and had given what comfort she had to offer.

Amanda, her emotional exterior growing thin in the last year, was not prepared for the 'visual' that medical technology had made possible. Tubes, I.V. lines, and sacks collecting drainage were either connected to him or making new orifices as the machinery hummed, keeping his lifeless body alive. His eyes were closed as she entered and the nurse, reassured that Amanda wasn't going to faint, squeezed her forearm and gave them their privacy.

"Eric, it's me...Amanda." She reached a gloved hand to clasp his. She was thrilled at the movement she felt in her hand. "I love you too." She knew he was conscious enough to hear.

Eric's parents and Mike one-by-one filtered in, all, with

the exception of Amanda, not knowing what to say or how to act. Most didn't use their allotted time and were ready to make an about face as soon as they entered. Physically and mentally drained, they gathered themselves, departed and went their separate ways, bringing with them silent torture that a situation like this can convey.

Amanda, alone with her thoughts, sat in the passenger seat of Beatrice's Toyota Camry. Beatrice, insisting she'd chauffeur this morning, was heading toward highway 101 to drop Amanda home. Beatrice, obviously losing an ample amount of sleep over the ordeal, began to question what Amanda planned to do once Eric returned home. "Will you tell Eric right away?"

"I'll cross that bridge when the time comes. Until then, I plan to take life one day at a time." Amanda's voice was a monotone.

Hours later, with sunset beckoning on the coastal horizon, the crystal, that hung from Beatrice's rearview mirror sparkled with dazzling colors. One beam of colorful refracted light bounced from Beatrice's watch and added to the images displayed on the disintegrating vinyl interior. Surprised that the late afternoon had arrived, she took solace in the fact that new hope would surely come with each passing day. Hope, for now, that Eric would muster the strength to pull through the whole ordeal.

The next weeks were crucial. According to the experts, telltale signs of success or failure would begin to surface within the first month. The hospital took no chances and the strictest guidelines were rigidly adhered to by all visitors and medical staff alike. Visiting hours were cut short for the first week. Most who visited were given the third degree and if considered an infectious risk, were asked to talk, with the aid of telephones, through the plate glass window that made up one wall of Eric's room.

Amanda, having not so much as a sniffle, came first thing in the morning and again in the later afternoon. Seventeen days had passed and, with the exception of some minor stomach upset, no signs of graft-versus-host had surfaced. Eric's spirits were higher than Amanda's, but she refused to let her distress enter the hospital. Today she stashed a one-pound box of See's candy in her bag.

Fully suited up, she entered and couldn't help but notice the vivid color glowing in Eric's cheeks. His respirations were deep and frequent. He smiled, hit the floor for a set of military push-ups, then came up for a 'breather.'

"Uh. . oh, caught by the warden. What will it be? Solitary confinement or should we go straight for the chair?" His voice was giddy and full of life. She loved him so much and for a instant, forgot their biological connection.

"For your information, it's lethal injection in California, and yes, for taking your chances with the harmful ecosystem on the floor, you will receive..." Thrilled at the life their conversation contained, she pulled the candy from her purse. "One box of nuts and chews to either be eaten quickly or securely hidden from the nurses."

He accepted the box, situated himself next to the candy so that he could converse, indulge and keep watch simultaneously. "You know the way to my heart." He stuffed one chocolate after another into his mouth, ooh-ing and ahh-ing with pleasure.

"I'm hoping you'll gain some weight." She couldn't help but notice how his shoulder blades protruded through the sheer hospital gown. She wondered how he was able to gather enought strength to do push-ups.

"Probably just increase my triglycerides!"

She closed her rubber-covered hand around his. "Did they say it was O.K. to work out?"

"Let's just say, they didn't say it wasn't."

"I see you haven't asked."

"If it was up to them, they would wait until hell freezes over, or my blood count becomes ideal, whichever comes first. Let's face it, when it comes to the benefits of exercise, the studies have only touched upon the tip of the iceberg. I'm feeling great, and the more I use my body, the stronger I'll become. Besides, the floor is probably cleaner than any plate you've eaten off of in the last month." He reached for another chocolate, but this time handed it to Amanda. "Here, you could use the calories yourself, skinny minny!"

Chewing, she managed, "You probably have a point. Don't worry, my lips are sealed."

❧

Less than three weeks had elapsed since the bone marrow transplant and Eric, half waiting for the torturous side effects, felt as healthy as a horse. Two nights in his own bed had done wonders for his emotional recovery. Visitors came often, but the bulk of his waking hours in the hospital were spent trying to drown out the moaning, snoring and humming machinery with the volume on his television remote control. His sleep went uninterrupted now and his days were met with an all-around better attitude. Amanda's care, catering to his every need, would surely be missed when he reached full recovery. His entire perspective had changed in the last months. He counted his blessings and appreciated all that touched his life that was good. At the moment the good he found was in the stack of buckwheat pancakes heavily soaked in maple syrup. His fresh ground coffee only complimented the savory breakfast.

Amanda joined him with a cup of coffee on the bed. "I see you are trying to fatten me up!" The words were hard to understand with the huge mouthful muffling his usual enunciation.

"You don't seem to mind." She watched intently as Eric devoured the stack, feeling like Mother Hubbard watching her brood. She loved to watch the nutrients go down and hoped that every meal brought him closer to a full recovery.

"I'm loving life Amanda. I feel great. In fact, I hope you will join me in a short walk this morning. I caught myself in the mirror and couldn't believe the ghostly image glaring back at me. The fresh air and mild sunshine should do wonders."

Amanda continued to sip the strong coffee and appreciated that she was able to give him a second chance on life. "I'd love to join you. I plan to monitor your every move. No running or I go straight to the doctor."

"You are no fun at all!" Eric paused after poking fun then changed his mind. "Well, except for last night."

THIRTY-ONE

One Month *Later*

Mona, accustomed to having intimate dinner parties of six or eight, had surpassed her entertaining capacity by at least thirty. Aware of her limitations, she had called upon the skills of topnotch caterers, known in many circles as Marin's finest. The mouth watering array of vibrant tropical delicacies were spread along the rented buffet tables. Mona supplemented the beautiful display with vases overflowing with fragrant herbs, handmade wreaths and colorful clippings, all fresh from her garden.

William, her son, pre-set the CD player on random play with soft reggae tunes from the Caribbean, some mainstream R & B, and the familiar rock-and-roll sounds of John Cougar Mellencamp, which had blared frequently from Eric's room when he resided at this address. The house, customarily dormant since Eric's departure, was bustling with life. A banner hanging over the fireplace read "Welcome Home Eric." On the elegant mantle and below on the seating area, gifts were piled high.

Seven weeks had passed since the bone marrow transplant, and Eric was recovering remarkably well. The subject of Eric's donor still hadn't been opened, aiding tremendously in Amanda's procrastination and hope that the subject would never be broached. It seemed the hospital had no intention of pursuing the issue either, and as time passed, the reality not only became easier to swallow, but easier to sweep under the rug.

Running always seemed to remedy what was eating her up inside, and she felt fortunate to have her favorite running partner beside her on the trail. They found themselves in the woods every chance they got. Amanda set a slow but steady pace, with frequent rest and refuel breaks along the way. Eric appreciated every moment, and his renewed approach to life was contagious. Tonight was a celebration of Eric's life.

Music reverberated from the living room and drifted into the backyard where Amanda caught her breath and sought out something refreshing to drink. Tiki torches adorned the perimeter of Mona's back fence and illuminated her beautifully manicured garden. Standing beside a huge yellow barrel filled with beverages and melting ice, Amanda was lost in conversation with William. He was a bit of a nerd. His homely wife watched the conversation like a hawk with unnecessary clean-up tasks, avoiding any and all social interaction. Initially, Amanda was sorry to have opened the topic of William's work. She was only being polite, and since he offered to open a new bottle of Kendall Jackson Chardonnay, she owed him more cordiality. He was flattered to have Amanda's attention, inserted the 'hooks' and rambled excessively, hoping his vast medical terminology would impress her.

Amanda nodded at the appropriate times as she glanced around the backyard for a prospective savior. The alcoholic beverages were refilled regularly by the caterers, and conversations were taken to the next level in the few clusters of people nearby, leaving Amanda on her own and bored to tears. Just when she felt trapped to the point of suffocation, the conversation took a turn. "...and my father knew the fertility clinic was a good deal when he saw it."

She immediately perked up. "Is this the clinic you run today?" She knew he was a doctor, but had never bothered to inquire about his specialty. It couldn't be...could it? she thought.

"Yes, it's one in the same." He seemed to be bursting with pride. "It's called Marin Fertility now."

She was hesitant to ask the looming question, and with

the stats pertaining to success rates of in-vitro fertilization that William was spewing, she was able to take a few deep breaths as she organized a tactful inquiry. "What a great success rate...It sounds as if you have changed the name." Deliberately opening the can of worms, she absorbed all he had to say, trying to control the pounding in her chest as he spoke.

"In 1957, my father bought the clinic, then moved it from Stanford to San Francisco. For a variety of reasons he didn't change the name. Last year, I moved the clinic to Marin and took the opportunity to change the name." William pondered his own greatness with a few deep breaths, then continued, "My father may have been a great doctor, but a risk taker he was not, I on the other hand—"

Amanda couldn't help interrupting, "So, the Clinic was originally called the Stanford Fertility Clinic?" Her breathing took on a pattern of its own and she began to feel lightheaded. She motioned to a nearby bench and took a seat. He followed without hesitation.

"Yes, run by a real quack, as my dad used to say, by the name of Dr. Welter. He ran the clinic into the ground, and when it had all but died, he fled to Florida with his secretary, leaving his wife and three children without a dime. A real asshole from what my father used to tell me."

"Is that why your father moved the clinic to a new city?" She knew she was prying and hoped all the questions weren't arousing any suspicion.

He leaned in and lowered his voice to a whisper. "Just between you and me," he said, proud to have such juicy gossip at his fingertips, "...my father seriously questioned this Dr. Welter's medical ethics." His eyebrows were undulating upon his brow bones, and William's wife had apparently had enough.

Close to six feet tall, she walked with a hunchback that was most likely the result of an insecure adolescence. She walked over to where her husband was sitting. "I think it's your turn to keep an eye on the kids. You know your mother will come unglued if they traipse through her garden." She was bitchy, controlling and wasn't mincing words. William immediately complied rather than face the firing squad later that night.

To smooth over the embarrassment and hopefully diminish later punishment, Amanda introduced herself to the Amazon, then turned to shake William's hand. "I really enjoyed talking..."

Trained to obey on command, William went to fetch the kids, without so much as a good-bye. Painfully, Amanda managed to converse with the woman until her neck literally could no longer handle the angle and her ears couldn't bear the constant negativity. Small talk remained on the surface and lasted less than five minutes. All the while, Amanda's mind remained on the topic of Dr. Welter and The Stanford Fertility Clinic—names she recognized and needed to confirm with Beatrice.

The hoopla lasted until after midnight, leaving Eric exhausted and slumped in the Lazyboy Deluxe in Mona's living room, while Amanda, Mona and Beatrice straightened up after the caterers had packed and gone. Amanda was happy Beatrice had asked to lend a hand, even with Mona's subtle hint for her to do otherwise. Mona, her hands full of empty cups and wine glasses, headed for the kitchen, leaving Amanda and Beatrice alone as they plucked the remaining soft drinks from the plastic barrel.

"I had such a wonderful time with your families and friends. That Sally, she's such the..." Beatrice's voice was sincere, but Amanda had to cut the compliment short to satisfy her curiosity.

"Beatrice?"

Aware of Amanda's tone, Beatrice stopped her train of thought, as well as her soda extractions, turned and gave Amanda her full attention. "Yes, dear?"

Amanda lowered her voice and double checked for privacy. "I had an eye-opening conversation with Mona's son, William."

"Oh, yes...nice boy, but that wife of his seems to be a bit uptight."

"Mona's son took over the Stanford Fertility Clinic after his father's death. His father purchased it from a Dr. Welter some thirty years ago."

Eyes opening wide, Beatrice commented. "Shortly after I left the clinic, I heard it was sold. I heard it was moved to the City."

"Yes, Mona's husband felt it was a good idea to move to the city and start with a clean slate, so to speak. According to William, the place was going under, sold for a song and Dr. Welter left for Florida with his secretary—Marcia wasn't it?—instead of his family."

"I always suspected there was more to their relationship than business." Beatrice, appalled at the notion, completely missed the point.

"I would love to look him up and give him a piece of my mind," Amanda said with intense conviction, bringing goosebumps over her entirety.

"It's not worth it...You can't let it eat you up inside. No sense looking back when you have so much to look forward to," Beatrice's said with true conviction.

"I know.. you're right.. but something inside wants him to realize the consequences I'm left to deal with because of his or his staff's negligence...or tampering, for all I know."

Mona, whistling an ancient show tune as she came down the back steps, halted their conversation. Delighted at the success of the party, she was oblivious to Amanda's tension. Mona had managed to find a place in her heart for Beatrice through the course of the evening and appreciated the extra hand she was lending. Picking up the remaining cups, she commented, "I just checked on Eric. He's sleeping like a baby in his old chair." Evident in Mona's expression was the fact that she loved him like a son.

"He had a wonderful time tonight. I haven't seen him move like that since the wedding." Amanda mimicked a few steps from the jitterbug.

"It was so gracious of you to throw a party, Mona. " Beatrice was sincere and Mona appreciated the sentiment.

"Oh, it was my pleasure. He lived with me for three years and helped me through a very rough time in my life. I think of him like a son, and I couldn't afford to lose him. It's like a miracle that he's afforded a second chance."

"Yes, it is." Beatrice looked Amanda in the eye and continued. "We have so much to look forward to now that he's recovering."

THIRTY-TWO

Thinking ahead, Amanda placed the calls from her office, eliminating the chance that Eric, or anyone else for that matter, would happen upon the phone bill. The office, usually immaculate and inviting, was piled high with uncompleted work, bids that she intended to pursue, in addition to a multitude of vases full of lifeless, decomposing flowers carted over a month ago from the hospital. Emanating from the wet foliage was a stench comparable to that of rank foot odor. Breathing through her mouth, she managed to ignore the awful smell for the time being.

With pad and pencil she dialed information for the Florida area and began her wild goose chase. The operator spoke in a slow southern drawl and politely referred to Amanda as "ma'am," making her feel old. Sue Ann, not busy and eager to please, retrieved from her computer screen several clinics, all of which had the word 'fertility' in the title and were located in the greater metropolitan areas of Miami, Tampa and Orlando. She was delighted to be of assistance and had every intention of looking at Jacksonville, Fort Lauderdale and Tallahassee if Amanda had no luck with her first list. Sue Ann doubted the existence of fertility clinics being located in the smaller cities, but encouraged Amanda to call her back if she had no luck reaching her 'friend' through the seven numbers she was able to retrieve from the computer.

Amanda, battling the idea of closing the book on her new-found knowledge, had decided to go ahead, without Beatrice's support. She realized full well that the whole idea of confronting Doctor Welter was not only preposterous, but was a means to no end. Nevertheless, she placed one call after another, inquiring about the doctor until, on the fifth call, she was able to zero in on his whereabouts.

"Good afternoon, Atlantic Fertility Clinic, how can I help you?"

"Yes, this is Amanda Edwards. I was wondering if a Doctor Welter works at your clinic?"

"Well, he used to work here. He ran the clinic, but he retired two, maybe three years ago. Why may I ask are you calling"

Amanda's brief conversation provided a wealth of information. Doctor Welter had apparently retired only two years prior. He and his office manager/wife had moved to Tampa to a well-to-do retirement village. The woman on the line had no problem voicing her ill feelings toward the Welter's incompetence, flipped through her rolodex, disclosing their whereabouts as of two years ago. She was naive and extremely gullible to Amanda's contrived story about her father and Dr. Welter attending medical school together years ago. From what Beatrice had told her, Amanda estimated the doctor to be in his late sixties to early seventies. The office manager swallowed the idea of a surprise seventieth birthday celebration for her father, hook, line and sinker.

At the close of their brief conversation, Amanda had in her possession the doctor's phone number as well as his address. All this, and it was only nine o'clock. Realizing the Southeast would be out to lunch for a while, Amanda took the opportunity to straighten the office and dump the putrid flowers into a Hefty bag, which she dragged outside, one step closer to the dumpster.

She couldn't help but feel foolish at her rather obsessive undertaking, but she felt compelled to forge ahead. She also felt some guilt in the fact that she and Eric had made love for the first time in months. She felt closer to him in some ways than she had ever felt before, but the truth was chipping away at her. She put in a CD to calm her nerves and decided to let the answering machine pick up the incoming calls for awhile. After all, in the past months she had been forced to refer the bulk of her clients elsewhere, some even to Henry, holding on to only the few who truly cared about her and had been sympathetic and patient through her personal ordeal. What's another couple of hours?...,she thought as she turned the machine on.

Melissa Etheridge sang with conviction and her contagious strength came through her lyrics, always making life seem a little bit easier. Amanda turned the music up and was taken in by the raspy vocals, bubbling with soul. She was on a roll, and actually enjoyed the distraction and change of venue from her customary 'married my brother' thought patterns. Removing the odor had improved the atmosphere at least two fold. A little air freshener, dusting, vacuuming, 'Windexing' and the office sparkled, making Amanda feel not only revitalized, but accomplished and ready to confront the 'enemy.'

Turning down the stereo, she took a seat and a simultaneous deep breath. Her hand trembled as she pushed the eleven numbers.

"Hello?" A soft spoken woman picked up on the first ring.

Clearing her throat, Amanda began her slightly rehearsed script. "Hello, I was wondering if I could speak with Dr. Norman Welter?"

There was a long silence then an inquiry. "Who may I ask is calling?" The voice was unsteady and timid.

"Amanda Edwards. Dr. Welter and I haven't had contact for over thirty-five years. I have some unfinished business to discuss. I was hoping..."

Before she could go into further explanation the shaky voice interrupted. "Norm passed away last spring."

Stunned, Amanda replied. "Oh, I'm sorry. . I, I really am."

No reply. More silence.

"Are you his wife?" Amanda's heart was pounding in her ears.

"Norm was my brother-in-law." Another long pause. "My sister was married to him."

Disappointed, but not ready to give up her pursuit,

Amanda continued the questioning, now walking on eggshells. "Is Marcia available?"

"Marcia...?" A moment passed. "Oh, you must be referring to his ex-wife. Norm, God rest his soul, and my sister were wed over twenty years ago."

"Oh, I see." Realizing her one last question was probably futile, Amanda went ahead in spite of it. "Oh, I see... You wouldn't happen to know how I could reach his ex-wife?"

"I'm afraid that she passed away five, six years ago. I remember my sister telling me about a card in the mail stating that the alimony payments were no longer necessary. They didn't even say how she died...I'm sorry."

"Sorry to have disturbed you."

As Amanda replaced the receiver, an unexpected, overwhelming feeling of relief swept over her. A load was lifted from her shoulders with the knowledge that Doctor Welter was no longer able to make mistakes with the frozen identities of unborn individuals. There was nothing more she could do, but she was proud of the fact that she'd had every intention of confronting the doctor responsible for her turmoil. She swivelled her executive chair and took in the view of the ocean. The Sausalito fog was just beginning to lift, unveiling a blue sky. A half dozen sailboats glided with the winds. She decided then to let it go and get on with her life with the man she loved.

Picking up the phone for a second time she dialed a familiar number.

"Braxton and Edwards accounting, can I help you?"

"Hi, Tina, may I speak to Eric?" Anxious to talk to his clients, Eric picked up the line before Tina had the chance to relay who was on the line.

"Hello, Eric Edwards here."

"For starters, the doctor said three to four hours maximum. It must be about time to go home and visit with the couch."

She picked up the portrait on her desk and touched his contagious smile.

THIRTY-THREE

Amanda's morning injections were a nuisance, but were a means to an end, and likely to bring much happiness into their lives. Besides, Eric had mastered the art and by the second week was able to inflict only the slightest of pain. The injections were composed of hormones that triggered the release of multiple eggs, rather than the usual single, readily available and mature and prepared for extraction.

Ironically it was William who initiated the idea of trying in-vitro fertilization, calling out of the blue from his clinic at Marin Fertility.

Luck was on their side when William and his team were able to harvest thirteen eggs. William, an extremely competent physician, was detailed in his explanations of the 'in vitro' process, as well as realistic in regard to the odds, making no promises. He preferred fresh sperm over the frozen he had to work with, but felt that Amanda's excellent health and her under thirty-seven status put them in the fifty percent range.

Artificial insemination, less invasive and expensive, was another route to be explored if the 'in vitro' was to fail, but William's offer to fully fund the thirteen thousand dollar endeavor, for a study he was conducting was one they couldn't refuse. A gesture of this magnitude, even if Mona may have prompted the whole idea, was the chance of a lifetime, and agreement came easily for Eric. Convincing Amanda wasn't automatic, but after a brief hesitation, Amanda warmed up to the idea. The fact that the baby would be closely monitored from the start and followed through the entire gestation held ample weight and convinced her to go ahead with the process.

William had available at his fingertips the best facilities medical technology could offer and, upon Eric and Amanda's request, had agreed to call upon a team of geneticists to analyze the embryos for any chromosomal abnormalities. Rest assured, Amanda would never give birth to an infant with severe defects again.

Amanda, feeling uncomfortable with the truth and guilty for not having the strength to tell Eric about the complications that might exist with a percentage of her pregnancies, longed for a baby with so much intensity and saw this as her only hope. How could she spoil Eric's dreams of being a father? Amanda thought. She went ahead with the plans.

Ten eggs were fertilized with Eric's frozen sperm and four of the highest quality embryos were selected and placed in Amanda's womb. This constituted their first try. The remaining embryos were frozen and stored for safe keeping if a pregnancy was not achieved.

The waiting began. Amanda attempted to go through her daily routine unaffected. Two weeks later at her appointment, William had disappointing news. He acknowledged her pain but spoke positively about successive attempts. She was instructed to wait at least one cycle, possibly two, before having the next set of embryos implanted.

THIRTY-FOUR

One Month *Later*

Nearly a hundred thousand people were gathered in a few square blocks near the Embarcadero—the makings for mass confusion on this foggy May morning. Adrenaline was in the air as Muni buses, stuffed beyond capacity, traveled toward the starting line. Ferries, leaving at the crack of dawn from other Bay Area locations, carted thousands, yet the bulk of crowd choose to risk insanity by carpooling in on their own. Hotels for six square blocks, booked solid weeks in advance, enjoyed the prosperous weekend, but had no problem turning down all who needed to use their 'facilities' on race morning.

The bus station was swamped, disrupting the homeless and degenerate, and the line for the women's bathroom was at least thirty deep.

Eric had run the 'Bay to Breakers' since college, always coming home the weekend before finals. He was still amazed by the elaborate costumes, which kept him entertained while he waited for Amanda. Thirteen guys from Hewlett Packard, dressed identically in blue shorts and logoshirts, tied the binding line at their waists that joined them into a centipede. All toted enlarged, Styrofoam computer chips on their heads, looking ridiculous and proud of it. The minority appeared to be runners, some weekend athletes, while most had the bodies of computer nerds and couch potatoes. The camaraderie and teamwork never ceased to impress Eric.

Every age group, race, religion, socioeconomic group

and athletic capability was present in today's extravaganza. A minority of three hundred were seeded and ran for the prize money and vehicle that would be awarded to the top male and female. For those individuals, this race, on the 12 kilometer course from the San Francisco Bay across the city to Ocean Beach, was competitive and fast. For most runners, the remaining 70,000 or so, the race was not so serious. They came to enjoy the event.

Every year, a fair share of runners abstained from costume — or any clothing, for that matter. In the early nineties a three hundred pound woman had strutted her stuff, turning many a head as she waddled her naked, cumbersome self, straining to breathe and perspiring up a storm. The majority cheered her on and were sad to see the news flash later that night indicating that she had been cited for 'indecent exposure.'

Engaging in the pleasures of voyeuristic activity, rather than placing any importance on the competition, Eric couldn't help laughing out loud when he witnessed a jogger wearing a Bill Clinton mask. Repeatedly the masked jogger claimed he had no plans of inhaling during the race.

Amanda wondered if relieving four drops was worth the long wait in the restroom line. The clock posted high on the cement wall read seven-forty. Just twenty minutes until the gun went off, and an additional ten to fifteen before they would move forward, and with luck, another twenty to run full out.

"It seems crazier than usual today." They stepped over some signs stating 'Transvestite Power' in bold red paint, en route to the starting line. "Oh," Amanda commented, "Can you believe those 'ladies' in drag were in the women's bathroom, adjusting their push-up bras and girdles and basically flaunting the illusion they intended to create."

"Only in San Francisco!" Eric reached for Amanda's hand, as the crowd thickened.

"Only at the Bay to Breakers."

With nearly two decades of experience under his belt, Eric

led Amanda up Howard Street, where the congestion was less claustrophobic. Howard intersected with Spear Street and put them in the pack, approximately thirty-five thousand back.

"Pretty good for seven forty-five, if I do say so myself!" Eric gloated as they pushed their way a little deeper, until the warmth of other bodies was enough to combat the morning chill.

"Oh, I can see we won't be stretching much before the gun." Now, more than ever, she wished her height hadn't peaked at five-three. She was inhaling only remnants of discarded air from those lucky enough to be blessed with taller frames.

"Believe me," Eric said. "The first two miles are an excellent warm up at the 'ripping' ten-minute mile pace."

Ten minutes to the start. The crowd's anxious excitement was evident in the flying tortilla Frisbees and beach balls, catching the air above the crowd. Will Martin, a weather forecaster from Channel 2, emceed the pre-race events and braved the masses as he stood exposed, high on a stage as he cheered the crowd and threw thousands of endorsement souvenirs. Basically, he set himself up as a human target for pre-race entertainment. Everything from sweatpants, food and jockstraps were aimed in his direction while he maintained a sense of humor and, hopefully, a hefty compensation.

Without Eric's persistence and frequent reiterating of the chemo treatments he endured, Amanda would be safely nestled in the quiet environment of their home. Not possessing the slightest inclination for such an extravaganza, this just wasn't in her nature. The failed pregnancy only added to her more introverted cravings. Pleasantly surprised, Amanda found the crowd to be entertaining and engaging.

Her only complaint was the fact that her height, combined with the sardine-like configuration, allowed less than ample amounts of fresh oxygen. Breathing in 'leftover' stale air left her feeling light-headed and in need of some quality oxygen. Eric, reading her mind, or at least perceiving her discomfort, crouched under her legs and scooped her up on his shoulders with one effortless motion. Out of surprise, she screamed, found her balance and rejoiced at the fresh air, as well as the much improved view of her congested surroundings. Taking several deep breaths, she made an honest attempt at feeling better. With the start approaching in less than five minutes, the crowd took part in a mass disrobing ceremony. Old sweats were tossed by the wayside without concern for where they might land. All participants were well aware that the homeless would find the gold mine and would be better off because of it.

The gun sounded and the seeded runners were off. Last year, shortly prior to his diagnosis, Eric was included in that pack; next year he planned to be there again. In the interim, he joined the masses and enjoyed the hoopla instead of the competition.

Forward movement occurred at roughly eight thirteen, prompting Eric to place his wife back on solid ground. Removing the 'ultimate' in sweat attire, which they had dug out of the archives of their closet, they began the trek towards the beach.

They had to maneuver carefully to hurdle the heaps of clothing without tripping. Thoughts of being stampeded were a great incentive behind this task. They watched the placement of each and every step.

They reached mile one at eight twenty-three. The crowd, still quite dense, began to thin, allowing for a slow jog if one were daring enough to weave through the pockets that began to develop. Helicopters, twin-engine planes and the Goodyear blimp toting various messages filled the skies. A cheering crowd filled the perimeter of the course. Many bodies fueled the excitement with music, dancing and outrageous costumes.

Camera crews were set up at every overpass and aimed to photograph all entrants wearing a race number. Every overpass was met with a flurry of waves and flailing arm movements from the runners with appropriate noises to match.

The real work began just after the two-mile mark at the infamous Hayes Street hill, a steep incline lasting a quarter of a mile. The crowd clogged once again, and the walkers were instructed to move to the right side of the course. Eric moved ahead and Amanda followed as she too, began to slow. Speakers set on the windowsills of the old Victorians blared soul music while the dreadlocked tenants danced, sang and encouraged the crowd upward and onward. The aroma of marijuana wafted from the open windows. At the top of the hill, the runners were met with a jazz band and the San Francisco Firemen in full uniform, saluting from their polished truck.

Looking at the masses behind him as he rounded the corner approaching Golden Gate Park, Eric expected to see Amanda trailing close behind. But she was nowhere in sight and he was disappointed, aware of the low probability of spotting her before reaching the meeting place they had decided on last night: the sign for the letter 'E' near the alphabetic display at the polo fields. With her recent runs faltering from her norm, combined with strict instructions from William to take it easy, she had no intention of holding Eric back from his all-time favorite event.

The fog began to dissipate, bringing warmth and sunlight to this beautiful May morning. The salty breeze off the ocean cooled Eric's face and body as it quickly evaporated his perspiration, giving him renewed strength and passion for the sport. His pace picked up, and he passed the familiar cluster running in his pack since mile two. Three naked guys were running in front of him, each sporting only a baseball cap. Eric chuckled as he read the inscription on the back of each cap. Buns—Of—Steel. The college-age men were probably on a dare but seemed to be having a good ol' time in spite of their nakedness.

Amanda had lost sight of Eric a couple miles back as he rounded the corner just past the jazz band. Her light-headedness persisted as a dull cramping sensation began in her gut. Where were the endorphins when she needed them most? Taking it easy, she anticipated feeling better at any moment. She stopped at the water stand and watched a few thousand pass. Plodding along again she began to feel weak, moved to the right and took it down to a walk. Unzipping her fanny pack, she extracted an apricot bar, inhaled it, and hoped it would help regulate her fallen blood sugar. If it weren't for the fact that the in vitro procedure six weeks ago had been followed by disappointment and her period, she would have sworn that she was experiencing initial signs of pregnancy.

Exhausted at the six-mile mark, she couldn't help but notice the commotion to her left, past the beautiful landscaping in Golden Gate Park. There was a huge gathering as thousands herded toward one place. She concluded it must be the polo field. In the center of the field, from what she could make of it, a band was setting up and practicing with the amps raging. Nearby, were tables stacked high with what she assumed to be race day t-shirts. Booths lined the perimeter of the grassy field where hordes clustered around to partake of the food, beverages and trinkets that were considered one of the perks at the finish line festivities.

Amanda, using the remainder of her fallen energy, merged to her left, cut across the steady stream of runners, maneuvered her body quickly and carefully to avoid tripping anyone, or worse yet tripping herself and being trampled. With only a couple hundred yards to go she found a path leading directly down to the field. She began to scout for the alphabetical display that Eric had described. She wondered if he would be there to greet her, or if she would be the first to arrive. She laughed out loud, thinking of the fun she could have with Eric, describing a totally fabricated story of the victorious day she had encountered.

The alphabetical display was placed around the perimeter of the booths with the "E" located clear across the field. With a few thousand people at each letter, the task of meeting up with a friend was minimized, but far from easy. With only twenty-six letters and close to a hundred thousand entrants, mulling over a few thousand can take some time.

She began scanning the bleachers set up behind the "E" as well as the group gathered in front of the sign, spilling partially on the field. Finding an open pocket, hoping she'd be more conspicuous, she continued row by row. Within a minute she heard a barely audible voice coming from a distance.

"Amanda, over here!"

She turned to see Eric jumping on the top bleacher, waving his arms wildly. She acknowledged him with all the vigor she could muster then waited as he took the bleachers two at a time. His color was vivid, his energy high and his shirt wet enough to wring out. He greeted her with a big squeeze that practically caused the regurgitation of the apricot bar.

"What's wrong, Amanda?" He couldn't help noticing her lack of color, and absence of perspiration on her face.

"My running really sucked today. I walked the last few miles and found a short cut to the polo fields." She pointed to the path across the field. "I thought once the crowd thinned, getting plenty of fresh air, I would feel fine."

"I'm sorry I lost track of you...I should have. . " Eric felt guilty.

"Did you have a good race?"

"Yes, but..."

"Yes, but nothing! You deserved to have a great run, Eric. This is your race and I wasn't about to cramp your style."

"Are you feeling O.K. now?...You look a little pale." He reached around her slight body to offer some support.

"Do they pass out barf bags at this race?"

"I think we should call William to see if the hormones were too hard on your system."

"I'm thinking along the same lines. Even my breasts are sore, and the light-headedness...I haven't felt right for a week. If I didn't know better, I'd think I was pregnant." Trying not to let her false hope build, she continued. "Do you think it's possible?"

"Anything is possible. Let's call William, and get to the bottom of this first thing tomorrow." He held her hand and they walked in the general direction of the Crystal Geyser station.

"Twisted french fries would really hit the spot right about now." Amanda scoured the booths in search of a way to alleviate her nausea.

THIRTY-FIVE

One Year *Later*

The dense canopy of trees absorbed much of the direct sun and gave the runners and hikers a reprieve from the heat as well as acting as a mobile for the infant riding in the stroller. The breeze intensified the skyward entertainment and was evident in the tiny feet that wriggled all the more whenever the wind picked up. The stroller experience was a first, but the familiar landscape and the sound of her parent's voices helped her feel secure.

Born a healthy baby girl, Beatrice Edwards defeated the odds stacked against her. She not only appeared healthy, but was free of any genetic abnormalities. Eric referred to Beatrice as the "miracle baby," and only Amanda and Beatrice Clooney divined a deeper meaning in the nickname. The truth about their biological relationship had tormented Amanda throughout the entire pregnancy, but ever since Bea's arrival, Amanda had grown to accept that Eric was her husband first and foremost. When, and if, the time was right she would break the news. For now they relished in their happiness and lived life to the fullest.

Beatrice thrived on the attention she received from her parents, grandparents and the numerous pleasing array of 'aunts' and 'uncles' who couldn't stay away. The most surprising metamorphosis came from Grampa Black. Amanda's father had a strong affinity for baby Beatrice and went out of his way to see his granddaughter, who bore a striking resemblance to him. He visited at least twice a week, taking time from his busy schedule to roll around on the floor, feed her and even change her diapers. Amanda was impressed by this side she wasn't accustomed to seeing, and respected the fact that he didn't even seem embarrassed at revealing his more feminine side.

Born with a soft-spoken temperament, baby Bea cried softly only before feedings and was inquisitive and content at all others times. She especially loved her front pack, where, depending on whose front she was adhered to, she could be counted on to be angelic for hours.

Moving swiftly up Eldridge trail in her newest mode of transportation, the infant took in the beauty surrounding her and cooed with excitement at the movement of the trees above. Eric pushed the jogger stroller at a swift pace while Amanda, challenged, kept up quite well. "Beatrice loves it!"

"She thinks the trees are one big mobile, propped here for her sole entertainment."

"Are we spoiling her, or what?" Amanda's breasts were huge and were harnessed down in an attempt to stabilize and reduce muscle tearing. The double "D" cups were equipped with easy access for breast feeding.

"We don't hold a candle to your father…I guess there was a good side buried there all these years." Eric slowed the pace as he could hear Amanda struggling with the conversation.

"At least Bea will benefit." She paused as she contemplated. "I didn't think it would happen in this lifetime, but I think there might be room for forgiveness."

"I'm so glad to hear you say that." He glanced back and couldn't help but notice her awkward voluptuousness. "Whoa, did you miss a feeding!?"

"No, but I am considering bagging my business and getting into wet t-shirt contests!"

Their laughter echoed through the ravine and Bea, sensing how lucky she was, wriggled her legs some more.

ABOUT THE AUTHOR

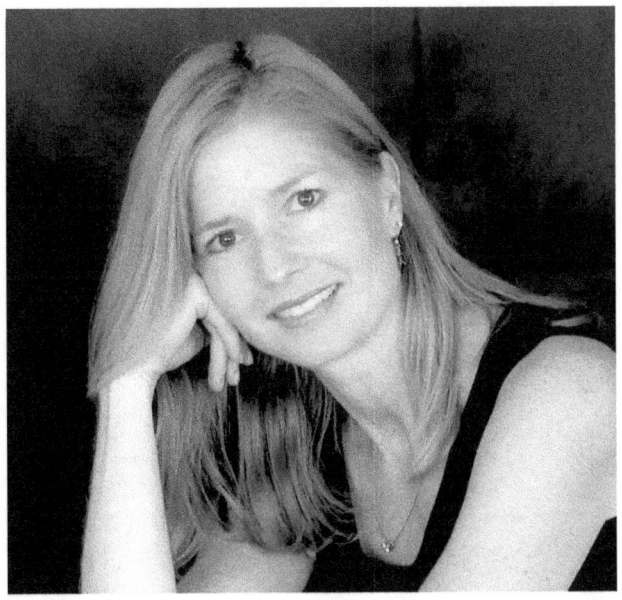

Karen grew up in Marin County, CA where her love to run and explore the hills and pastures was nurtured by Marin's natural resources. She left to pursue a degree in exercise physiology and returned seven years later, married and ready to embark on her carrier as a health educator and begin a family. Karen's passions include running, reading, writing and photography but most significant in her life is her family. Along with her husband, Steve, Karen has two daughters, Whitney and Madison. They are her true jewels.

www.ingramcontent.com/pod-product-compliance
Lightning Source LLC
Chambersburg PA
CBHW071410170526
45165CB00001B/232